Betty Bethards

The Dream Book

Symbols for Self Understanding

Other books by Betty Bethards:

Be Your Own Guru

There Is No Death

Sex and Psychic Energy

Techniques For Health and Wholeness

Way To Awareness

Seven Steps To Developing Your intuitive powers
(AKA: The Way Of The Mystic)

From My Heart To Yours

Betty Bethards is a widely known lecturer, author, mystic and spiritual healer. Because of her down-to-earth approach and infectious sense of humor, she is affectionately known as "The Common Sense Guru." A popular radio/ TV guest in the USA and England, she has written nine books and has made 29 audio cassettes.

Before becoming the innovative, approachable teacher that she is, Betty was a housewife with four kids. And then her dramatic death experience shattered her belief system and values, and led to her discovery of mystical and psychic abilities. Soon after, Betty founded the Inner Light Foundation which provides ongoing lectures, seminars and workshops in holistic health, spiritual development, interpersonal communications and other human development areas. Long before doctors recommended meditation to their patients, Betty's was a lone voice, showing people the many healthful rewards of the practice.

Through her *The Dream Book*, Betty has shown how amazingly easy and beneficial it is to understand one's dreams. More than 300,000 people now own *The Dream Book*. An international Best seller, the book is published in 9 languages.

See Betty online at www.Innerlight.org. The Inner Light Foundation address is: P.O. Box 750265, Petaluma, CA 94975, telephone number: 707 765 2200, Fax: 707 765 1939, Email: Bettyilf@aol.com.
Ask for a newsletter.

Betty Bethards

The Dream Book

Symbols for Self Understanding

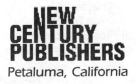

NEW
CENTURY
PUBLISHERS
Petaluma, California

Library of Congress-in-Publishing Data

Bethards, Betty
The dream book: symbols for self-understanding/
Betty Bethards -- 21st ed.
p.com.
LCCN: 2001130283
ISBN: 978-0-918915-03-0

1. Dreams. 2. Dreams-Dictionaries. 3. Dream
Interpretation. I. Title.

BF1091.B47 2001   154.6'3'03
                        QB101-200278

Cover design: Montanesque Enterprises™ (www.montanesque.com)
Cover concept/copy: Charles Rubin Advertising
Cover photograph Copyright © 2003 Russell Illig/Getty Images
Author photograph: Mary Ann Halprin

Printed in the United States of America
21st Edition
Fifty-fourth Printing

NewCentury Publishers
P.O. Box 750265
Petaluma, CA 94975
Tel: 707 769 9808
Email: Newcentpub@aol.com
www.NewCenturyPublishers.com

Distributed by SCB Distributors

Contents

This book is lovingly dedicated to my daughter, Pam, whose enthusiasm for working with dreams awakened me to their importance in daily living.

Preface

Betty Bethards is widely known as a psychic, mystic, spiritual healer and meditation teacher. Her publications, lectures and media appearances have helped millions of people in their search for self-knowledge.

Betty began lecturing and giving seminars on dreams when she realized that "dreams are your greatest tool for understanding yourself and your life." But most people neglect this free inner resource of guidance.

"People have been asking me for this book for years," Betty explains, "and at long last here it is. I have channeled information on every symbol in the book, which as you can imagine was a time consuming task. But I learned so much in the process! Now I gladly share this with you."

Betty's channel is her attunement to her higher self, spiritual guidance or God self. It is a vehicle for receiving insight and information which is usually beyond the reach of the conscious mind. She is quick to point out that everyone has a channel, a level or frequency of awareness called higher consciousness. Attuning to it is really listening to the teacher within or your own guidance. She believes we are particularly receptive to this level in the dream state.

Betty explains that dreams are her most treasured source of knowledge, because the conscious mind cannot get in the way to distort their message. "You can learn to remember your dreams, recognize their meaning, and use them for inspiration and problem solving," she teaches. "They tell you what you are doing right and how to change what needs to be changed. Since we spend one third of our lives in the sleep state, it is certainly to our advantage to use this time for insight."

The Dream Book, Symbols for Self-Understanding, is divided into two parts. Part I: Self-Understanding Through Dreams includes three chapters: The Meaning of Dreams, Working with Dreams, and Dreams and Expanded Consciousness. Part II: Dream Symbol Dictionary lists more than 1600 of the most common dream symbols with cross references. You are encouraged to read Part I before using Part II.

Betty points out that it is "not necessary to accept my philosophy to use this book. You may be an atheist, agnostic, or have some sense of a universal mind or higher power. But no doubt you do recognize that you use only a small percentage of the mind. Learning to work with dreams enables you to develop more of your mental potential."

Remember that you are your own final word in dream interpretation. If the suggested meaning does not *feel* right, keep exploring until the sense of the meaning resonates within your own being. You can always check a good dictionary for possible additional clues. Also, different symbols have different meanings depending upon your life experiences and association with the symbol. In dream interpretation as in every other phase of living, be your own guru. Learn your key symbols and then it is easy to begin deciphering specific messages.

May this book inspire you to begin and continue exploring the wise and wonderful world of your dreams.

PART I

Self-Understanding Through Dreams

CHAPTER ONE

The Meaning of Dreams

What's In a Dream?

Are dreams some strange, mysterious phenomenon that spontaneously happen on the night shift of life? Or is there some deeper meaning behind this universal experience?

Throughout recorded history humankind has valued the dream. A source of guidance, inspiration, prophecy, prediction and problem solving, dreams are a common experience to us all. They know no boundaries between young and old, rich and poor, races, religions and nationalities, In every culture we find some version of "sleeping on a problem" before making a decision. The Bible and other ancient texts are filled with examples of how dreams have played important roles in people's lives.

What is this wonderful dimension that is so near and yet so far? To understand the real meaning of dreams we must delve beneath the surface to the *purpose of it all*. Why are we here? How are we to answer the age-old question: Who am I?

We Are Interdimensional Beings

Dreams begin to awaken us to the fact that we are spiritual

or interdimensional beings, *in* the third dimension, or time-space, but not *of* it. They are like a letter from the higher self to the conscious mind. They awaken us to higher resources of knowledge within ourselves, giving us information on what is happening in our daily lives and how to meet and move through the problems that face us. Dreams also give us information on the future, so we are forced to ask, "How could I know a thing like that?"

A dream helps us realize that we are here only temporarily on the stage of waking reality. What we call life is really a school. There are many schools or levels of consciousness in the universe, and earth is one of the most important. During our sojourn here we are learning more about the true nature of our beings. We are learning that we are infinite creative energy or love energy, and that all of our hurts, disappointments and disillusions come from a failure to recognize this truth of who and what we are.

The name of the game is growth. In all our experiences we either *go* through or *grow* through them. If we just *go* through them, then we will repeat them again and again until we learn the lesson behind the appearances. If we *grow* through them, we are free to move on to the next step in the learning process. But to understand more about the game of growing and learning, we will look at two age old concepts: karma and reincarnation.

Karma and Reincarnation: Lessons and Learning

The interwoven concepts of karma and reincarnation were hard for me to swallow coming from a fundamentalist Baptist background. But as I learned more and more through my channel I began to realize they made a lot of sense. These ideas have been known in both eastern and western traditions since early times, and once had wide acceptance in the early Christian church.

Reincarnation suggests that a person is basically spirit or consciousness which takes on bodily form and is born lifetime after lifetime. Reincarnation is the natural, normal process of the evolution of the soul. The soul is the etheric or energy body, the eternal part of our beings. It is neither male or female, but an integration of energies. You have layers or energy bodies within the soul which you shed as you go to higher levels of spiritual awareness. At physical death you shed the earth body as a coat, which is the lowest of the energy vibrations.

Once you have learned your lessons on the earth plane, having gained balance mentally, emotionally, physically and spiritually, you then go to the celestial plane and live in a much higher energy level.

Each soul chooses how fast it wishes to progress. Between incarnations and in the dream state at night one receives teachings. When the soul returns to earth, to time-space awareness, it brings back knowledge and training and works to put it into practical application while in the body. Each being designs a plan for growth before an incarnation, what it hopes to achieve in that lifetime, what karma it wishes to work out. The soul is free once it incarnates to go ahead with the plan or change its mind. Your teachers, of course, are going to be there encouraging you to get on with the program. But you are free to do whatever you want to do with an incarnation.

Karma refers to the law of cause and effect which governs one's experiences over collective lifetimes and within the individual lifetime. Karma means as you sow, you reap. It is the principle of individual responsibility which underlies all the teachings of my channel.

To effectively work with dreams we must recognize that we control our own destiny through our thoughts, words and deeds. We have to relinquish our martyr and victim mind sets and accept responsibility for what is going on in our lives. Then we will benefit from dreams as a tremendous teaching source.

Chance of a Lifetime

Because of your past karmic ties and awareness of lessons to be learned, you intentionally have chosen the circumstances of your present existence. Before you ever incarnated you knew what the first 28 years of life had in store for you. You chose your parents, sex, race, nationality, socioeconomic conditions, astrological sign. Whatever your circumstances, you set them up. If you chose anything less than a perfect body, it was for a reason: never to punish, only to teach. There is *no accident or coincidence* in life. Nothing happens by chance. Everything we perceive of as suffering is really a wonderful opportunity to correct past mistakes or imbalances and move toward our ultimate goal of enlightenment.

Once we get the idea that we have created our own situation here in the earth school, we are able to ask why. What is my positive lesson? What is this teaching me? Then at last we stop blaming others for our unhappiness and realize no one can limit our lives. We cannot change others, but we can change ourselves and move beyond any given situation. Every relationship and every experience is nothing more than an opportunity to grow through limitations.

Self-Love as Karmic Key

Karma follows you from your very first incarnation and continues throughout all succeeding lives. As you sow, you reap. What you build you have to pay off. Some souls wait two or three incarnations before they face former ties. But if you handle situations with love and awareness, you not only will transcend your karma, but you will also free the other soul. It is in forgiving that you are forgiven.

The message of karma, in fact of all the earth plane existence, is learning to love yourself. As you fully love and honor the God within your own being, you fully love and honor the God within all beings. You can then never hurt self or another soul.

All of our lessons evolve around self-love. To love self you must go beyond ego identification and attachments. The true self is the spiritual energy within, the creative power behind all forms. Love is the absence of fear, and fear is the last great illusion that separates us from inner truth.

Most dreams are showing you fears and limitations that you imposed upon yourself; they help you recognize the importance of facing your fears. As you do, you discover a deeper level of insight, beauty and joy within.

You are free to create your own heaven or hell on earth. But it is just as easy and a lot more fun to create your own personal paradise to share with others.

Dreams and The Death State

My channel has explained that the only difference in the death state and the dream state is that the silver cord, which is much like an umbilical cord connecting the soul with the body, is severed in death. This cord allows the spirit to travel in realms and planes beyond the physical at night, and to receive higher teachings. As you go to sleep at night, and your consciousness leaves the physical body, you are experiencing the same thing as death. As you gain more and more control of the dream state you will realize that there is no such thing called death as we are taught to believe. There is no death, only a change of awareness. Gaining more control of dreams enables us to realize that we truly are interdimensional beings. The life energy, or God, is the changeless medium of being which underlies what we call "life" and what we call "death." God is the medium of all experiences, levels and energies. Eventually you begin to identify with the eternal nature of your being, rather than the stages you are going through or the particular level of consciousness in which you happen to find yourself.

Dreams and Cycles

We go right along with nature in our cycles of learning, growth, resting and integrating. We have yearly and monthly cycles, not to mention the seven-year cycles of changing into something completely new.

Dreaming follows the natural cycles of growth during the year. From spring to fall you are in an accelerated period of learning. Your lessons are coming very fast, and the energy is heightened. You will be given teaching dreams that show you when you are missing a lesson. But it is more difficult to remember dreams during the spring and summer months unless you are programming and working with them.

When the energy of the fall begins to mellow out in October, November and December, the dream state will not be as predominant. You are unwinding, integrating the lessons of the busy growing season.

The winter months are usually when you have the clearest and strongest dreams. This is your spiritual or inner growth time. Whatever lessons you did not learn from spring to fall will be back next spring. You are being prepared for the next growing season and are being shown all the things you need to work on. During the winter your inner schooling is intensified. You will be more apt to remember dreams even if you are not working with them. The winter is also seed planting time. You are getting ready to blossom into spring. This is a time to set your goals for the spring, ask for insight, and determine your path.

Dreams are also affected by the lunar cycle. Five days before a full moon dreams begin to get stronger and clearer, peaking with the full moon energy. If you are not centered, the full moon can scatter your energy and your dreams may seem strange. You may become depressed during a full moon cycle, or experience energy fluctuating to extremes. Again, the more centered and in control of your own life, the less you are affected by outside influences. Instead, you are able to use all energies to your advantage, inviting them to heighten and awaken you to new understandings rather than getting thrown off base.

Understanding Self as Energy

Dreams often show us which energy centers or chakras are out of balance. If you are being stabbed in the heart, for example, you are losing energy from the heart chakra. You may be getting too involved in other people's trips and empathizing with them instead of seeing how they set themselves up for a great learning experience. Or you may be giving love energy to a partner and not getting any back. It helps to pay attention in dreams to the area of the body that is highlighted, and understand the accompanying lesson.

To understand chakras we first must recognize that we are energy beings, systems of interpenetrating energy fields. We experience ourselves as male and female in bodies, but this is a very limited perception of who and what we really are.

There is one life energy, or God force, whether you call it the Holy Spirit, universal mind, psychic energy, sexual energy, love, or *kundalini*. I use the term *kundalini* because that is how I have been taught by my guidance.

This *kundalini* or life force is housed in all of us at the base of the spine. This is our infinite reservoir of spiritual energy. When we begin to direct it to higher energy centers of our body, we begin to expand our consciousness and recognize that we are spiritual beings.

There are seven basic energy centers or *chakras*. The word *chakra* comes from the Sanskrit term meaning *wheel*. Clairvoyants who perceive these finer energy dimensions of the human system see each chakra as a spinning wheel of energy. Although this has been part of the Hindu tradition for centuries, only recently have we in the West become more fully acquainted with it. We are beginning to recognize, for example, that acupuncture and mastery in the martial arts are built around an understanding of the power and flow of these forces within.

Chakras correspond roughly as the etheric dimensions of our endocrine glands. The soul, or etheric body, is connected to the physical body through these centers.

The chakras provide us with the key to understanding ourselves as expanded beings. The centers are located in the base of the spine, sexual organs, solar plexus, heart, throat, between the eyebrows (third eye) and the crown of the head. There are many focal points of energy within the human system, but these are the major ones.

Each chakra represents a way of understanding ourselves and the world, a way of perceiving reality. If we suppress or block energy at any of these levels, disease will manifest in the corresponding area of the body. Different diseases will manifest as a result of blockage in any given chakra depending upon an individual's mental and physical makeup. Also, if a chakra is too wide open disease may result, for we would not have control over the amount of energy flowing through it.

Our health depends upon a dynamic balance of energy among all the chakras, plus a balance of the male and female polarities within. We must learn how to awaken and direct energy through our systems to maintain maximum health and well-being.

It is important to realize that all of the chakras are open to a degree, but we tend to operate out of some more than others. In each individual one or two will be weaker than the rest, and it is in the weak or blocked ones that tension or disease will manifest. Emotional suppression, for example, will manifest as disease in the area where there is the least energy—a blocked chakra—and then can spread to other areas. Cancer, a result of suppression, manifests behind whatever chakra is blocked. This can be a result of tension, fear, negative thinking, or sitting on your own unhappiness and not making changes. It is the end result of your lack of awareness. The key is to open the system, cleanse and flush out the energy field with the natural healing processes, and release the negative thought patterns that are responsible for the disharmony in the first place.

The Root Chakra. The life energy or kundalini is housed at the base of the spine. The first or root chakra serves as a trigger to release this energy.

In the first chakra there would be no energy blocks. The first is like a storage bank for the kundalini. The kundalini comes up naturally twice in our lives, once at puberty and again at menopause. At puberty when the kundalini is activated it is bringing the entity into the awareness that he or she is a particular physical vibration, and the male and female chemistry comes into alignment. In addition to the heightened sexual awareness, however, it is also a time of creativity.

Again at menopause, which both men and women experience, the kundalini kicks up as another chance to use this life energy to renew your physical, mental and spiritual being. A hormonal change is involved for both men and women. The energy often gets stuck in the second or sexual chakra, and people choose to have what they call one last fling before settling into old age. But if the energy was truly understood, it could be transmuted into a higher level of vigor and well-being. It certainly should not signify that we are going over the hill, but rather that we now have a heightened creativity which can propel us to the most creative and productive time of our lives.

These times of puberty and menopause are stressful due to the changes taking place, but through an understanding of energy and the practice of meditation they can be heightened periods of growth which open the door to continued vitality.

But ideally we learn to trigger this energy from the root chakra whenever it is needed, to use it to maintain a high level of awareness at all times. The important thing to remember here is that it is always with you as an infinite reservoir of vitality and strength.

The Second Chakra. The second or sexual chakra is the first that can be blocked. Suppression of energy here may result from fears and guilts about sex, feeling inadequate in one's sexual role, having sex infrequently, being in a bad marriage, feeling unfulfilled in love and sleeping around, holding on to unpleasant memories from previous relationships, or trying to lead a celibate life and not understanding how to channel the energy into higher centers.

The suppression is expressed as violence, explosions of anger, prostate or female organ problems, colitis, and other physical ailments in the lower abdominal region.

It is important to utilize and release the energy in the second chakra in some way, whether through masturbation, a creative outlet, sexual intercourse, meditation, or a combination of these. It is vital that we get in touch with our sexual needs and determine whether we are blocking energy in this center.

The Third Chakra. The third chakra or solar plexus is the area in which most people experience their difficulties, particularly sensitive people. This is what I call the worry chakra. It is a very vulnerable center.

If this chakra is not balanced or is too wide open, a person will pick up everyone else's trips, whether positive or negative. One will experience extreme nervousness, and may find gall bladder problems, ulcers or other stomach problems.

To balance this chakra one needs to learn how to detach from other people's trips, which is best done through building the energy in meditation, getting more physical exercise, and using the energy in some creative outlet. When this center is balanced it can serve as a valuable intuitive guide, for then it is no longer swayed by fear and anxiety.

The Fourth Chakra. The fourth chakra or heart center s the first of the higher creative centers. This is the center of the Christ spirit, or unconditional love for oneself and one's fellows. It is a beautiful level through which one experiences unity with all life. But it has a dual problem.

First, if it is too wide open, you will pick up all the suffering and the pain of the human condition, being unable to detach and gain a perspective on it.

This has always been one of my biggest problems: I will be so aware of your hurting that I will be out there trying to clear it up for you, rather than seeing how you set it up and what you are learning from it. This leads to playing the mother-counselor or father-counselor role, which is very safe. It is all right to play that some of the time, but we also need to work with someone in a one-to-one relationship in which we become vulnerable enough to look at our own numbers.

Second, if the heart center is closed or walled off, you will be unable to love yourself and others. Being walled off in this center not only blocks you from being sensitive to another's feelings, but may result in high blood pressure and heart problems. (We build up and carry around many resentments and hurts here, overloading this area with unnecessary tension.)

The ideal is to be open and channeling energy from this center, but perceiving from the more objective third eye chakra.

The Fifth Chakra. The fifth chakra is associated with higher creativity and clairaudience (psychic hearing or perception of finer vibrations), and is easy to block through tension. Blocks here manifest most readily as tension in the back of the neck, often resulting in backaches, headaches and eyestrain. Rheumatism and arthritis are a direct result of blockage across the neck and shoulders. Throat problems also result from suppression in the fifth center.

Other blocks are caused through lack of verbalization of one's real needs and feelings. Expressing your creative ability, communication with yourself and others, are important to the proper functioning of this center.

The Sixth Chakra. The sixth chakra, also known as the third eye, is not a contributor to much illness. If a person has been concentrating for long hours he or she may experience a buildup of tension between the eyes, resulting in sinus headache or eyestrain, although usually this is a result of blockage in the fifth. The third eye merges into the crown or seventh chakra after a person has been meditating for awhile, and the two are as one center.

The third eye is associated with the opening of true mystic potential and spiritual knowledge, seeing with the one eye of truth. When one has learned to direct energy through this center it can be a powerful healing beam, stronger than a laser.

The Seventh Chakra. Also known as the crown center, the seventh chakra represents union with the God self. Pictures of saints and religious teachers often show a ring of light around the head, seen by poets, artists and clairvoyants, which is the emanation of energy from the merger of the sixth and seventh chakras. This center is not associated with blockage and disease.

The Purpose of It All

The purpose of it all, is to know yourself and to see all

lessons as positive opportunities to learn and grow. That sounds easy enough, but my guidance always did like to keep things simple. We have come to earth to learn and each of us has free will and must find our own way. What we seek is within us. Although we were not handed a manual of living when we were born, we were given teachers who walk with us.

No one goes through this trip alone. Each one of us has a guardian angel and a team of teachers who guide and support us along the way. These wise and powerful beings do not make our decisions for us, but lead us to insight so that we can make our own wise choices. We would not want others, whether in or out of the body, to make our decisions because then we would not learn.

Three Free Tools

The most valuable tools for helping us along in life are free and available to all: dreams, prayer and meditation. If we would take advantage of these, much of the guesswork, confusion and hardship of life would vanish.

Dreams. Dreams, of course, are the subject of this book. They give us a daily reading on what is happening in our lives. They provide a door to the superconscious mind for insight, problem solving and higher teachings from the other side.

Prayer. Prayer often is misunderstood as a valuable inner tool. Many people see prayer as a means of appealing to a whimsical higher deity, begging God for things, hoping that they will be granted. This kind of orientation toward God belongs in the Dark Ages.

God has given each of us the creative power to manifest whatever we want in life. We already have all the richness and love of the Divine Spirit within us. God already knows what we want, and "it is the Father's good pleasure to give you the kingdom." The key is that you have to know what you want or you are not going to be able to manifest it. Prayer, then, is the formulation in your mind of what it is that you want or need.

Prayer means getting very clear within yourself. It is stating what you feel would best help your growth and awareness at this time. You may ask your higher self to direct or guide you into making the best possible decisions for yourself, but remember it is you who must choose.

Prayer often is best expressed in the form of positive affirmations, such as: The perfect career opportunity opens for me now. The natural state of my being is health, harmony and wholeness. The power of God flows through me, strengthening and guiding me. The perfect relationship is manifesting in my life now. I am being divinely guided and directed in all that I do.

You may have heard people say that prayer does not work. It works if you understand what you are doing. In the law of mind, like attracts like. If you affirm and feel love and wholeness, you bring it into your life. If you affirm prosperity, you invite it to dwell in your consciousness and affairs. Most of us ask for things out of a feeling of fear and separateness, rather than acknowledging our oneness with God and our divine birthright as spiritual beings. We ask for things having no real sense that it is within our power to create them, to bring them forth. Whatever we create within must manifest without.

Also, doubt and feelings of unworthiness, the "I don't deserve" number, often surround our prayers and we undermine our own efforts.

To effectively pray, relax and get very still within yourself. Fill yourself with a strong sense of love, wholeness, power and attunement to God. You may wish to repeat affirmations, such as, "There is but one Presence and one Power, God, the Good. I am relaxed and at peace in this inner Presence. All things are working together for my good. The spirit of God is active in me now, and I formulate clear goals which lead me to the expression of my highest good. Recognizing the power of God within me, I now ask for or affirm . . ." and then state your prayer.

When you pray, especially if for things, opportunities or a particular relationship, always remember to add: "This or something better." The rational mind too often is attached to specifics. The ways of higher mind, or God, are indeed beyond the understanding of our everyday consciousness. There may be a wonderful new dimension or opportunity awaiting you that you have not yet thought of, but that will be brought into your life if you are but open to receive it. Prayer is never to be used in a manipulative way, or you will get absolutely nowhere. It is useless to pray that someone else change to meet your expectations, or that someone else love you. Avoid trying to run other people's lives through prayer. We can send others light and love, but must honor and release them to use it as they see fit.

Love, opportunity, joy and abundance await us, but they may not come through the specific persons or situations we had in mind. We must be willing to release ourselves and others into God's care, trusting that we will find what we seek, and that all things are working together for our good.

Prayer, then, is a way of focusing your conscious mind on goals and life direction. It is honoring the power of God within you to support and actualize desires which are for your highest good.

Meditation. Meditation is the freeway to enlightenment. It helps us get in touch with the teacher or God within. It opens us to higher energy sources and recharges body, mind and spirit. Perception depends upon our energy level, and meditation is the way to keep energy at its highest.

Although positive changes are experienced immediately

from meditation, many are gradual. You will experience a reduction in stress and tension, an overall improvement in health, and feelings of peacefulness. But meditation is not a wonder drug that relieves all ills overnight. It begins to sensitize you to problems at hand and maintain your energy level, so you are better able to deal with whatever is facing you. It gives you the eyes to see and the ears to hear, so you can see how you are getting out of life exactly what you feel you deserve—nothing more, nothing less!

The meditation I teach was given to me by my channel. It is an ancient Egyptian method and is one of the fastest and easiest. Actually, there are two parts to the total process. First is concentration, a directed mental effort that precedes meditation. Concentration quiets the mind and consciously focuses it on something. Second is meditation during which you relax your mental focus and allow a free-flowing reception.

This technique requires about twenty minutes a day. It is best to meditate when you are alert, rather than right after a big meal or when you are very tired.

You may find the early morning hours best, so that you can heighten your energy and orient in a positive way before beginning each day. Or, you may rather meditate right before going to sleep. This will help you clear out the clutter from the day and raise your energy so that you are more receptive to the teaching dreams you are given. But any time is better than no time, and whatever best suits your personal schedule is what is best for you. But it should be a time when it is quiet and you will not be disturbed, as loud noises can be quite jolting in the middle of meditation. Before you begin you might spend a few minutes reading something inspirational, such as poetry, religious writings, or perhaps listening to uplifting music. This will help you tune out of your everyday concerns and get ready to meditate.

I include this meditation technique in all of my books,

and it may be summarized in seven steps:

1. Sit in a straight back chair with spine erect, feet flat on the floor. Your back should not be touching the chair. Fold your hands together in your lap, or hold them in a prayer position. Hands must be touching. Eyes may be opened or closed.

2. Take several slow deep breaths, and feel yourself relaxing. Imagine a bright white light completely surrounding you, which is your protection as you open sensitive energy centers.

3. Gently concentrate on a single idea, picture or word for about ten minutes. Select something that suggests peace, beauty, or a spiritual ideal; or just listen to soft, soothing music. If using music stay with the melody and words for the full twenty minutes.

4. If your mind strays from your object of concentration, gently bring it back to your focal point. (Surprisingly soon you will find your ability to discipline the mind growing much stronger.) It takes twenty years to still the mind totally so do not get discouraged. It works in spite of us.

5. After ten minutes separate your hands and turn them palms up in your lap. Close your eyes if opened.

6. Relax your hold on the concentration object, and shift your mind into neutral. Remain passive yet alert for ten minutes. Placidly observe any thoughts and images as they may come and go. Just be still, detached, and flow with whatever you are experiencing.

7. After ten minutes do your affirmations and visualizations as you are now at your most relaxed and centered time. Then close your palms, and again imagine that you are surrounded by a white or gold light. Now open your eyes. The light sends love and healing out to others yet buffers their stress/tension from influencing you as you go about your daily activities.

This twenty-minute period, however, is not our only practice. We should endeavor to practice the meditation attitude, watching our thoughts and behavior, throughout each day. Meditation can thus help us to be more fully involved in life because we can watch how we set up our experiences. Sometimes the changes are dramatic and sometimes they are subtle. But meditation does change your life because it changes you.

If you are meditating regularly, clearing each day as you go along, asking for insight to problems, you will not need as many dreams to show you what is happening in your life. You will already know. You will see how you are setting yourself up. Also, you will gain a greater sense of clarity on life goals and directions which can be formulated and manifested through prayer.

The dream images and the meditation images are the same. Until you get very clear and objective, however, it is still quite easy to allow the conscious mind to get in the way of insight you receive during meditation. That is why the dream state is much more reliable until you have been meditating for a number of years and can recognize the difference between conscious desire and genuine intuitive direction.

CHAPTER TWO

Working With Dreams

How to Remember a Dream

Everyone of us can learn to remember dreams. This, of course, is a prerequisite to working with dream symbols. After you are reliably recalling dreams, you can begin to program them for problem solving.

The most effective way to work with dreams is to keep a dream journal. Date each entry as you go along, for you will begin to see patterns and recurring themes as the weeks go by. If you do not understand an important dream message, you will be given more dreams trying to get the same point across. So do not worry about losing a big lesson; you will be given the message again and again until you finally get the idea. The most important thing in learning to remember a dream is your intent to do so.

Before going to sleep sit on the side of your bed (if you lie down you may fall asleep before you finish the process), take several deep breaths and relax. Then say to yourself, "Tonight I *want* to remember a dream and I *will* remember a dream. As soon as I awaken I will write it down." Then go to sleep with a pad and pencil beside your bed, *expecting* to remember and write down a dream as soon as you open your eyes. If you prefer, record your dream in a cassette tape recorder.

When you awaken, whether at 3:00 a.m. or right before getting up the next morning, immediately record any impressions, images, or feelings about the dream. If you do not usually remember dreams, you may have only a vague sense about it: a feeling of frustration, uplift, concern, peace. Just write down whatever you sense in the waking moment. If you have good recall of most of the dream images, put down everything in as much detail as possible: people, vehicles, scenery, objects, colors, shapes, numbers and so on.

If you do not immediately write down the dream, you will lose it. Do not think that you can go back to sleep and remember it later. You are in an altered state of consciousness, that half-awake half-asleep state when you first open your eyes. Until you learn to build bridges between levels of consciousness, you will not be able to recall your dream once you are fully awake. That is why you tell yourself you will remember *and* write down the dream.

By continuing to practice this technique of writing down material, bringing it back from superconscious to conscious mind, you are learning to bridge the gap between levels of consciousness.

You dream all during the night, but often your best teaching dreams occur between 3:00 and 5:00 a.m. or right upon awakening. Of course, if you are working the night shift and sleep during the day, your dream schedule will be adjusted to your biological rhythms. But dreams can come at any time whether during a nap in the afternoon or a catnap after dinner.

Using Dreams for Problem Solving

Even if you do not consciously use dreams for problem solving, you no doubt have had the experience of waking up in the morning with a clear and simple answer to a problem. You may not even remember a dream, but you know what to do in the situation at hand. This technique has been used for centuries to get insight. The conscious mind can struggle and wrestle with a problem, but when it is released to the superconscious mind, the greater infinite resources of consciousness, the answer effortlessly appears.

Deliberately programming your dreams for answers to problems, however, is taking even more control of the dream state and letting it work for you.

To use dreams for problem solving, again sit on the side of your bed before going to sleep. Take several deep breaths, relax, and bring the problem to mind. Whether it concerns relationships, career, health, inspiration for a creative project, or whatever, go over in your mind all the different parts of the problem that seem relevant. You have already thought about it, reflected upon it, but you are not sure which is the best direction, or the most positive solution. Feel into the problem as well as mentally reviewing it. Now mentally repeat, "Tonight I will have and remember a dream containing information for the solution to this problem. The problem concerns . . . (and briefly describe it as objectively as possible). I will now have this dream, and will recall, understand, and record it upon awakening. I open myself to the highest possible insight and guidance." Then go to sleep, completely releasing the situation from your mind, resting in the expectation that you will receive the answer.

As soon as you awaken write down everything you can remember. Write down any general sense of the dream, feelings, impressions, as well as images. You may awaken with a clear recall of a dream which, upon analysis, gives a very definite answer. You may awaken with a strong sense of just knowing what to do. Or, sometime during the day, something in waking reality may trigger an image or impression from the dream, and you have your answer.

You may recall a dream that you cannot seem to figure

out. Just record it, and continue the process the following night.

Avoid telling yourself that the process is not working, however. It is working; you just do not yet understand it. So if you do not have the answer you want upon awakening, do another little relaxation before starting your day. Suggest to yourself: "I have completely released this problem or situation to a higher wisdom within me. This answer is now presenting itself to me. I am open and receptive." Then dismiss the concern from your mind. Holding on to it or worrying about it will block your insight. If you do not get the answer during the day, repeat the programming procedure again before going to sleep. You should have the answer to any problem within a three day period.

Some people have said to me: "But I have tried to program dreams and it just did not work." There may be a variety of reasons. First, anything that affects the chemistry of the body significantly—alcohol, drugs, barbiturates, Valium, sleeping pills—may completely botch dream recall. Your dreams will not be clear if you are able to remember them at all. A full meal right before going to sleep also affects dream life in a negative way.

Second, it is important to be relaxed when programming or asking for a dream. Do deep breathing and relax your body. Still the conscious mind enough to focus on the programming technique. Feel the desire to problem solve or get insight from your dreams. Don't just mouth the words. You want the feeling of the heart center but the detachment and clarity of the third eye, so you are not reacting emotionally. Love yourself for creating the situation. It is a valuable teacher. Love yourself for now desiring to resolve and move beyond it. Love all persons involved for helping you learn and get to know yourself. When you approach problem solving through love, the answers are more readily available to you.

Third, ask yourself, "Do I really want to know what is best? Or am I trying to dictate the answer? Am I really open to the best and highest solution, or am I blocking my receptivity through fear?" Sometimes we ask for things that we really do not want to know. Particularly if the problem involves a decision over a major transition—leaving a relationship, changing jobs, taking self-responsibility—we may not really want to hear it. Ask, and you shall receive. But the asking must be an honest, open asking.

Finally, you may not be asking the right question. Questions should always have to do with insight into self, not how to change or manipulate others. If you are asking how to get your spouse to stop drinking, you are starting in the wrong place. Instead, realize that it is his or her responsibility to change, and all the love and support in the world may not be enough to help. The question should be: why have I created this situation for myself? What in myself needs to be changed to enable me to have a love-filled, joyous life? Through a need to be needed, a martyr syndrome, poor self-image or a number of other things, you may feel stuck in a situation. You can be assured of only one thing: with genuine self-insight the situation will change. You may have to leave it, you may not. But above all you must desire wisdom, not limiting ideas about self and others.

Remember the greatest thing we can do for another is to honor his or her inner power to make decisions and choose the kind of life he or she wants to live. We are all free to make our own mistakes. That is the only way we learn. When you are too concerned with shaping up someone else's life, you can be sure you are copping out on your own lessons. If you are saying to yourself, "If so and so would just change, then I would be fine," that is handwriting on the wall that you are avoiding self-responsibility.

So, ask for insight into self. Release others to learn their own lessons. You certainly can pray for others and send them love. But do so in the way that you are honoring their higher self, giving them the energy and freedom to make their own decisions, to determine their best life path, whether or not it may include you and your expectations and desires.

Kinds of Dreams

There are six basic kinds of dreams, and often you will remember snatches from several of them. As you begin to work with dreams more and more, you will recognize the differences and determine the value each is offering you. I call these different dreams clearing house or clutter, teaching, problem solving, precognitive, prophetic or visionary, and outside interference.

Clearing house. These dreams clean out the input from the day, sorting through mental and emotional clutter, rerunning experiences. Often the mind is still running a mile a minute when you first try to go to sleep. You are worried, anxious, stressful. These dreams begin the process of releasing useless concerns and integrating helpful ones. They help body and mind begin to relax.

If you meditate before going to sleep, stilling and focusing the mind, the clutter dreams are usually unnecessary. If you practice briefly rerunning the day in your mind, blessing, releasing and forgiving self and others, you are ready for a higher level of awareness in the dream state. Also, your energy will be higher and your dreams will be clearer.

Teaching. You usually have one important teaching dream a night. This gives you information on problems you are facing, or shows you higher teachings from advanced levels. You are prepared for what is going to happen during the next 24 hours. Often a *déjà vu* experience is remembering what the superconscious mind stored in the subconscious memory back during the dream state. You already knew you were going to say something in a certain way, or that a particular person was going to do or say something. Most dreams are concerned with what you are presently going through and how best to deal with situations and relationships.

You may find yourself sitting in a classroom, giving or hearing a lecture, or walking with a teacher in some beautiful surroundings. You may be hearing information you never knew before and have good recall of it upon awakening. Many discoveries and inspirations have come from higher levels of these teaching dreams.

Problem solving. These are dreams you have programmed or asked for. You may be seeking insight on understanding a difficult relationship, solving a scientific mystery, or asking for the plot of a new novel. All knowledge and information are available to you when you learn how to tap it. Learning how to program dreams and understand their messages is one of your most valuable inner resources.

Precognitive. This dream gives you a glimpse of something in the future. It is different from the *déjà vu* experience, because precognition is usually concerning someone other than yourself. Precognition means foreknowing. There is a special sense or feeling to the precognitive dream. As you learn to recognize it, you will know which images are symbolic and which may happen to be literal precognitive events. It is a psychic level phenomenon.

Most precognitive dreams are given to awaken people to expanded dimensions of the mind. Often non-meditators will have them, for then they are forced to ask how they know such and such about a particular person. The mind, of course, is not bound by time. Hopefully these dreams direct your attention inward so that you become more interested in developing and learning about the inner self.

Prophetic or visionary. This dream comes from the highest level of the soul. It is a message from God or the God-self and concerns spiritual growth. It comes from the mystical level of awareness. It may have a personal message or may contain a universal truth. The vision is on a much larger scale than what you commonly associate with dreaming. It has a totally different quality of awareness about it. You know you are awake, aware, yet also realize you are in the dream state. Prophesies of old and mystical teachings have come through the visionary level of consciousness. A vision has many qualities within it: insight, understanding, expansion, realization of the oneness of all life, power and love. I may have only one vision a year, but it is always worth waiting for.

Outside Interference. This dream is produced when something in your physical environment is causing enough disruption to get incorporated in your dream story. For example, you dream you are very hot and awaken to find too many covers piled on top of you. Ringing phones, barking dogs, cold feet on your back—anything can be a part of the dream, with no real message from the superconscious or higher self.

Also, if you fall asleep watching television or listening to the radio, any or all of that information can affect your dreams. It is always best to sleep in a quiet, restful environment. There is enough blaring into the subconscious throughout the day without adding more to it during your sleep time.

Indigestion or a full bladder also affects dream images. Just be aware when interpreting dreams that you may be picking up such outside interferences.

Anatomy of a Dream

Dreams often present themselves in three steps. First they give the time reference for the problem, situation or program you are running. For example, if you are shown a house you lived in when you were a child, the house represents an old program or awareness of self that started way back then.

Second, they will show you how the problem is manifesting now in your life and present awareness—what is surrounding it.

Third, they will present the solution to the situation, or how to learn from and move beyond the program or problem that is limiting you.

Most teaching dreams will follow this format. If you remember seeing a car, house, school or person of your past, that is usually part of the first phase of the dream.

Understanding Dream Symbols

The most curious thing about dreams, perhaps, is they speak to us in symbols. These may seem strange, but once we understand the meaning they are much clearer than our usual way of attempting to communicate with ourselves and others.

Why, you may ask, do I have to go through all the symbology in dreams? Wouldn't it be easier just to get the straight message? Communication among people is difficult at best. So many things are open to misinterpretation because of blocks and perceptual filters.

My guidance has said that dreams are given symbolically because once you know your own symbols you cannot mistake the message. You will know instantly what is being given to you and you will understand it totally. Actually symbols are like shorthand and are much easier to interpret than verbal conversation.

Working with dream symbols might be compared to playing the piano. When you first begin you are certain that this has to be the most awkward and complicated thing you have ever undertaken. But after a routine of regular practice, your new skill becomes a natural, flowing easy part of your life.

Or, take the computer industry. If you do not understand computer language, it all seems foreign and difficult. If you hear someone speaking a language different from your own, it is the old "It's all Greek to me" feeling. If you speak, read and write Greek, however, it is another story.

So think of working with dream symbols as just learning another language. They are a higher, more accurate, more integrative level, that enables you to become aware of self as an interdimensional being.

The Starting Point

There are primary dream symbols which usually have the same meanings. A good place to begin is to realize that everything in the dream is you. You are the producer, writer, actor and director. People in the dream usually represent qualities within yourself you have projected on to them. Male and female figures represent your own masculine and feminine energies. A child represents your child part, an aged person an old part of self, either one that is wise or a part that is dying because you have outgrown it. Animals represent feelings you have about specific animals or the characteristics associated with them; for example, a wolf is danger, like the wolf in sheep's clothing; a fox is cunning and craftiness.

A house, building, store or other structure is you. If it is large, it indicates great potential and awareness of opportunities and/or inner resources. If the rooms are cluttered, you obviously are not keeping your house in order. If some of the rooms are dark, they are parts of the self you do not know or understand. The attic or upstairs represents the spiritual self, the ground floor the physical or everyday self, and the basement the sexual or subconscious self. The various rooms and how they are decorated and arranged indicate that particular aspect of your life; bathroom—cleansing, eliminating, releasing; dining room—nurturing, fellowship, and so on.

Any vehicle—a car, plane, spacecraft, boat—also represents the self. It is your mode of traveling or being in the world. A car is your physical vehicle and indicates how you are traveling in everyday life. Going backwards, downhill, the wrong way? Got a flat tire? Are you speeding ahead in perfect control? A boat or ship is your emotional vehicle and lets you know what is going on in your emotional life. Are you being tossed upon the seas of life, going up and down? Are you in dry dock? Are you at the helm? Do you have an anchor?

An airplane or any airborne vessel is your spiritual vehicle, and if you are on your way to the airport, you know you are preparing to take off to new spiritual understanding.

A motorcycle or bicycle means you need balance in your life.

Water represents the emotions, fire is purification, air is the spiritual self and earth is the physical self (or degree of grounding).

Once you begin to recognize a few basic symbols, then you begin to look for colors (you do not dream in black and white), clothes, people, scenery, objects, sizes, shapes, numbers, words, letters and so on. Everything has its own significance. Fences or road blocks indicate that creative thinking is needed to get beyond a particular problem that is now facing you. The kind of road on which you find yourself traveling represents how smooth or rough your journey is at present. If you are on a freeway it is easy going. If a bumpy road you are getting there but it is a little rough at present. If you are paving a road you are making your way easier for the future.

Any symbols given to you—whether in fantasy, meditation or guided imagery—are all the same. They are coded messages from self to self. When you "get the picture," you understand the situation.

You Are The Final Word

Remember that you are always your own best interpreter. You are the final word on the meaning of a symbol for you. Do not be so gullible that you eagerly accept another's interpretation. This is giving away power and neglecting the refinement and trust of your own inner resources. If the symbol in the dream dictionary does not feel right, look it up in an unabridged dictionary. Often meanings are there you have never considered before, and a little bell will ring in your head when you read one of them. The definitions offered in this book are generalized and if they do not apply to a specific situation, you need to keep looking, reflecting, and meditating upon a symbol until it reveals its true meaning to you. And by working them out, they become so simple that you know you are always being guided by your own higher self or the God within you.

Common Types of Dreams

Nothing is off limits in the dream state. We are open to experiencing all levels of self, all fears, frustrations, suppressed images, unknown territory, visionary insights. We will become more comfortable with all dream images when we learn to welcome them, whatever they are, as symbolic messengers of self.

There is no such thing as a bad dream symbol. The most grotesque or frightening dreams have the most positive insights once they are worked out. Remember, dream images are just trying to get your attention, so do not resist them. Seek to recognize the insight so you can move on to more joyous awareness. Many people have the following common types of dreams:

Nightmares. A dream known to most all of us is the nightmare. It is one of our most valuable teaching dreams because it shows us a fear that has been blown way out of proportion

or something we have suppressed that is affecting us negatively. Often we do not remember the happy dreams. But the
frightening ones will make more of an impression and we
will be more inclined to work them out.

For example, a man had a recurring nightmare that a large
rat was eating away at his neck. He would awaken screaming
and clawing at his neck to remove the rat. Upon analysis, he
discovered that the neck represented the throat chakra. He
was not verbalizing his needs, and the suppression was
gnawing away and resulting in self-destructive behaviors.
The rat was an insecure part of self that was betraying him.
We must always nurture the inner self, taking care to verbalize and express what it is that we want and need. After he
began to take assertive steps to resolve problems both at
work and in his personal relationships, the rat dream no
longer continued.

Disaster Dreams. Whether earthquakes, flood, fire or tidal
wave, a disaster indicates a sudden change in some area of
your life. A flood means an emotional upheaval and an
earthquake means a big rearrangement in your affairs. They
usually indicate turning points or opportunities to take advantage of a new direction. See specific disasters in Part II.

Sexual Dreams. Sex is a big part of many dreams, and usually has little to do with the literal meaning of intercourse.
Usually it indicates learning to balance the male and female
polarities of our being. Remember that each one of us is both
male and female, manifesting in a particular body.

To have sexual intercourse in a dream represents a merger
of energies. If having intercourse with a man, it is a merger
of masculine energies within the self; with a woman it is a
merger of feminine energies. If you are a female (or male)
and dream of making love with another female (or male)
you actually know, it represents taking within the self qualities you associate with the particular individual. Making love

with a member of the same sex usually has nothing to do with homosexuality.

Also, having intercourse in a dream with members of your family does not indicate a desire for incest. If making love with your father or mother, it represents a merger of wiser, nurturing qualities of the masculine or feminine self; with a son or daughter, an integration of the more childlike or youthful qualities of self. Remember all persons in the dream are an aspect of you.

A sexual dream accompanied by an orgasm may indicate a need to release and balance physical energy, and this is a way the body has of restoring equilibrium. We must remember that we are physical, sexual beings and this part of the self needs to be honored.

Costume Dreams. If you find yourself in a costume, it usually represents a past life. It may be that a problem you are facing now was the same you were dealing with in another time and place. Remembering and understanding the dynamics of the costume dream will help you gain a perspective on whatever is presently confronting you.

Direction Dreams. The direction in which you are traveling indicates whether you are on the right track. If you are going up in a dream—up a mountain, up a road, ladder, staircase, elevator, whatever, you are going in the right direction. If you are going down, it is the wrong way. If you are going both up and down, your energy is scattered and you need to get centered. Going around in circles speaks for itself. If you are going to the right, you are following the path of intuition and guidance. To the left is the intellect and reason.

One man asked if he should participate in a conference and got a dream showing him riding on a down escalator, so steep that he had to heave his briefcase in front of him in order to hold on. Wrong direction, not in support of his study and projects at hand. Another example: a woman was considering the purchase of a certain automobile. She was shown the car sitting down at the bottom of a hill, and she had to walk down crowded streets to get there. She did not buy the car, and a much better offer came up within a few days.

Flying. Flying dreams are great fun, and usually mean you are consciously out of the body. If you can gain control of a flying dream you are free to go anywhere you like. You may think yourself in different places in time/space and instantly be there, or you may transcend dimensions. If you are flying around and then start losing altitude or think you are going to crash, it simply suggests that you have a fear of exploring higher dimensions and breaking out of limits. Try again the next night.

Falling. If you dream you are falling, you are probably having a bad landing coming back into the body. We all leave the body at night. If you jerk as you are dozing off, it is a bad exit. If you wake up and cannot move or talk, it means you are half in and half out of the body. We cannot move until we are totally in. Think yourself down to your feet. This will ground you.

We leave the body at night, or transcend physical awareness, to be taught and trained. The physical or third dimension is illusion; the dream state is reality. Through meditation and working with dreams you will never fear death as you will experience the fourth dimension and be as comfortable there as you are in the third dimension here.

Obscene Dreams. Nothing in a dream is obscene once you understand the meaning. Nothing is meant to insult you or offend you, but to get you to look at a level of self or limitation that you have avoided. Work it out and usually you will find a great deal of humor behind it.

Recurring Dreams. Like a movie rerun, there is a message you are not seeing. Recurring nightmares mean that you have not dealt with a particular fear. Recurring fence or barricade dreams mean there is a limit you imposed upon yourself that you have not yet recognized and removed. These are most important to write down and work out. Once you get the message they will stop.

Snake Dreams. Snakes frequently appear in dreams, and are power symbols. They represent the kundalini energy, or life force. One woman dreamed that a snake entered her lower body and moved up through the body trunk to the throat. The snake stuck in her throat, and she started choking. She awakened horrified. At first glance this does seem a bit unnerving, but actually it was a perfect explanation of what was happening in her life. The kundalini power is housed at the base of the spine. So the snake enters her body and begins to move upward. As we awaken energy it moves up through the various chakras. Her energy was flowing well until it reached the throat center, and there it stopped, causing choking. She was blocking energy in that center, and not verbalizing her needs and feelings. She was choking off communication because of fear and a poor self-image. This dream explained that her inner power was alive and well, and through releasing the blocks in the throat center by verbalizing and not suppressing she would get past present limitations in relationships with others.

Money Dreams. When you dream of coins or dollar bills, it represents changes coming into your life. Small coins, small change. Lots of bills, big changes.

Toilet Dreams. These dreams concern how well we are taking care of our inner garbage. Are we letting go of unneeded thoughts and experiences? Are we releasing the past so that we are able to live fully in the present? Difficulty in elimination or constipation indicates suppression. Diarrhea suggests forced elimination whether ready or not, and we are out of control in the process. A stopped up toilet means you are not releasing, flushing out negativity and wastes.

I had a dream with three stopped up toilets sitting out in the open. This was letting me know that I had to clean up my act mentally, physically and emotionally. I was now aware of things to do, priorities to establish, because the toilets were totally exposed for all to see.

Blood and Guts Dreams. Blood in a dream means loss of energy. If you are being stabbed, note the area of the body and check the corresponding chakra to see how you are losing energy. If you are being murdered or are murdering someone else, you are killing off a part of the self. This may be an aspect no longer needed, or a part that you are failing to nurture that is still valuable to self growth.

Death Dreams. A death means the ending of the old and making way for the new. A death seldom means a literal death. Rather it suggests the dying of a part of self necessary in the process of growth and regeneration. It may also mean you are dead inside and need to awaken feelings and sensitivity. So check carefully the symbols in the dream to get the message.

Chase Dreams. If you are being chased, or trying to run away from something, you are avoiding looking at a problem. If you cannot get your legs to move or are moving in slow motion, you soon will have to confront the fear you have been avoiding. When you are being chased, you are putting yourself through unnecessary anguish and pain. Remember to turn around and confront whatever aspect of self is chasing you, make peace with it, and the drama will end.

Dream Interpretation

Dreams may come in almost any form and use any symbol or story line imaginable. Recognizing the feeling level in the dream as well as the particular symbols is important to understanding its meaning.

First, write down the dream as fully as you can. Second, write down all the symbols you can identify and the possible meaning beside them. Look them up; check an unabridged dictionary if necessary. Third, write out your interpretation.

The following is a sample dream and its interpretation:

Step 1: The Dream. A *woman* was on a *bus* with a *spiritual leader* and members of a *spiritual group*. A *man* got on the bus wearing a *dark coat* and *hat*. He started *robbing* everyone. The *woman* had *$600* in her *wallet*. She was *lying* in a *sleeping bag*. She wanted to hide her *wallet* but her *left hand* was asleep and she could not move.

Step 2: Recording dream symbols:
woman – feminine, creative part of self
bus – large vehicle for growth
spiritual leader – her own higher self, spiritual teacher
spiritual group – growth conscious parts of self
man – masculine, assertive, strong part of self
dark – the unknown
coat – cover, hiding
hat – role she plays
robbing – stealing energy
$600 – 6 is your guidance, higher teachers, White
    Brotherhood (teachers of light); pay attention
wallet – identity
sleeping bag – in a cocoon, hiding in a womb
left hand – receiving hand
asleep – numb, passive, not allowing others to
    give to her.

Step 3: Interpretation: The feminine part of the woman has a large capacity for growth. Many parts of herself are growth conscious and she is with or being led by her higher self. She has covered up or suppressed the strong, assertive part of herself. It is unknown to her. She allows people to take her energy without ever saying no. She gives her power away. The 6 is her guidance saying: look what you are doing. Be assertive!

She is afraid of losing her identity by being assertive and she is unable to do anything about it zipped up in her cocoon. She is unable to receive and allow others to give back to her. All her energy is going out, not returning. Her inability to receive is the main message of the dream.

Levels of Interpretation

A dream can be seen on many levels. There is a literal meaning which is usually not the correct interpretation. But it depends upon what you ask for.

For example, a woman asked that she be given insight on her marriage. She had tried many things to improve the situation, suggesting counseling, communication, and so on. In her dream she was shown herself and her husband in a desert, walking up to a trader selling phony wedding bands made out of tin. When she looked at her husband, his face was in a haze, distant. When they rode out of the desert and stopped at a little house for refreshment, she was greeted by a stranger who embraced her with a warmth and love that she immediately knew was missing in the relationship with her husband.

This dream could be interpreted that her masculine and feminine parts of self were not balanced, but she had asked specifically about the relationship. In this case the woman was working on balance within. As much as she did not want to hear it, she realized the relationship was not based on mutual love. It was not really a marriage, and no growth (desert) symbolized its present state. The series of dreams which followed indicated the same thing. She knew then that she had to leave.

This was a positive solution to the problem. Although

some of the answers we receive may not be what we want to hear, they are always for our highest good. As soon as the woman was out of the relationship, she wondered what took her so long to see the situation and get on with her life.

Working With Dream Images

All dream images have a symbolic message. The ones that are the most startling are the fear images. We have many fears we have suppressed from childhood on, and these are free to surface in both dream and meditative states. It is important to remember that you are not your fears. Fears are simply negative thought forms which have no reality on their own. When we take away their power, they no longer have any influence over our lives.

Although our purpose in life is to meet the self, we spend a lot of time running away. We are afraid of many things, especially those which are unknown to us. We fear that which we do not understand. Each fear represents a block to our true beauty, the inner spiritual being. We should welcome all these frightening images, as they will reveal to us limited thinking and beliefs that thwart our development.

Any images that you identify but do not understand can be met and worked with in a "do it yourself" guided imagery or through meditation. This technique is particularly helpful when working with frightening images. If you have a frightening monster creature, or a frightening person, it is a fear blown out of proportion. Upon awakening bring the image back to mind. Imagine this "being" unzipping its monster costume, letting the fearful outer garb fall to the floor. Instead a little part of the self walks out, maybe a tiny little person, who offers you a present. You ask the little being what it has to teach you and imagine it lovingly giving you its message.

You can establish a dialogue with any dream image and let it talk back to you. Just do a Disneyland number with it.

If it is a tree, imagine it with a face, arms and legs, and ask it questions. If it is a big fence or wall, again, give it a face and let it talk to you. Imagine what it would say. To use this technique effectively, try the following steps:

1. Write down a description of the dream image you do not understand.
2. Relax, enter a meditative state, then picture the image in your mind. If it is inanimate, give it a face and let it talk to you. If it is big and fearful, imagine it unzipping its scary Halloween suit and stepping out as something quite harmless and ordinary. Then strike up a conversation. Remember, the scare tactics are just to get your attention.
3. Now ask: What insight have you brought me? Or, What part of myself do you represent? Allow the image to speak to you; make up what you think it will say if words do not come readily. You may actually hear words or just get a strong sense of what this form really represents.
4. After the conversation, thank the image for appearing to you. If you still feel unclear, ask it to present itself in a different form in your next dream so that you will understand.

When you begin to gain control of the dream state, that is, when you know you are dreaming, then you can stop and meet images while still in the dream. If something is chasing you, you can turn around and say, "Hey, wait a minute. Let's get this thing settled. Why am I allowing you to chase me, and what part of me do you represent?" When you can confront an image in the dream, you get immediate insight on what it is. And as soon as you face a fear, you have conquered it. Keep a sense of humor and you immediately restore perspective.

Also, when you become aware at any time you are dreaming, you can stop a dream and say, "All right, now I am ready to learn." You can ask any question and the answer will be given. This is what we are working to do: to gain complete control of the dream state so that it becomes a vehicle for higher learning and integration of self.

CHAPTER THREE

Dreams and Consciousness

Link to Enlightenment

Throughout our existence we are striving to integrate levels of consciousness within us, for then we will know no limits in awareness. A dream helps us begin to bridge these levels: the conscious, subconscious and superconscious minds.

The conscious mind perceives space-time reality through the five senses and is the rational or intellectual level. The subconscious is like a storage bank which contains all experiences in this lifetime, both in and out of the body. The superconscious goes way beyond. It is like the God-self, or higher consciousness, that is totally detached and watches what is going on. It understands completely the life purpose and soul mission. It is from this level we are able to get in tune with our whole life plan.

Dreams are your direct link to God, higher self or guidance. Although all knowledge is available to us, we cannot have instant enlightenment. We must be able to stay grounded and utilize information as it is given, incorporating it into our lives before going on to the next step.

My guidance has explained: "There is no instant enlightenment. You want to be very sure that you are grounded as you are opening up to higher levels of awareness. By getting insight through dreams and applying it in your daily life, you begin to integrate understanding. You realize that you are completely responsible for your own life and have no right to inflict your will upon another. As your insight expands, you earn the right to move on to the next level. If all instantly were given to you, you would not know how to use such power and knowledge."

Dreams and Self-Knowledge

Dreams help you see yourself as you are: your true inner beauty, your potential, where you are both missing and getting the point of lessons you are working on. Nothing is more important than to know yourself. This makes all things on all planes in all realities easy.

My channel has explained, "You do not have to suffer to grow. This is not what God intended, not His concept at all. It should be delightful to learn to know yourself. You all are going to make mistakes, and some things will seem awkward and uncomfortable at first. But if you can go out as children with eagerness and curiosity for learning, you will begin to understand what a wonderful adventure living really is.

"Nothing is unchangeable. When you dream of a particular problem or situation in your life, remember it is given to you in order that you may creatively resolve and move beyond it.

"The most difficult program to break is viewing change as something frightening, difficult, painful, or a lot of hard work. If you want to make life hard on yourself, this is your choice. God is patient. There is an eternity to learn that living is joyous and effortless. You create your life daily. You can choose to change it at any time. When you tire of running from lessons, you can make joyful progress very quickly.

"The key thing is to have the eyes to see and the ears to

hear. Some people have this when they incarnate, others take longer to develop it. This is the ability to sort out truths from all teachings, experiences and people around you. Lessons are being presented to you constantly, whether through your own or someone else's life. You can learn a great deal by watching other people interacting with one another. Watch and observe, but do not judge. This is the key with both self and others."

Gaining Control

When you begin to gain control of dreams, you are often aware when you are dreaming. If you are being confronted with fears or strange images, you can ask them what they represent and will immediately get the answer, as I mentioned before.

Through gaining control of the dream state you are able to raise your awareness to higher and higher levels. The higher your energy, the greater your awareness, the easier your life is. You become much more attuned to creating what you want, and begin reaping the benefits of your true birthright, which is joy, abundance, understanding, wisdom and love.

Use it—Don't Lose it

The biggest problem in living and learning is that people will not consistently use the tools they have been given. If you go to the trouble to program a dream, get insight on a problem, and do not implement it, what is the use of all the bother? Life is very simple, but we must ask, receive, recognize and implement. The follow through is the big one. Having the courage to trust the inner self, to act on our inner convictions, opens us to freedom and full self-expression. Remember that you are the architect and builder of your life. You can have great plans, but the daily work of construction and implementation is what gets the job done.

The conscious mind or waking state is really our time for home work. It is the time to practice the lessons, to put the insights to work. It is not goof-off time. Many people who have been meditating or watching their dreams for years with no apparent change in their lives can discover the reason is quite simple. If you spend twenty minutes in meditation, or ten minutes writing down a dream, and then do not watch the negative thinking and self-destructive habits of living the other twenty-three plus hours, you have achieved little.

Dreams and meditation give us the lessons and principles. Waking reality gives us the creative opportunity to practice using them. To grow and change we need to *integrate* insight into our lives. We need to practice, practice, practice.

The irony of it is that we create all the situations in our lives to teach us things. We set ourselves up for lessons, and when they come along we feel hurt. Self-pity means you need to be aware of your illusions. The very hurt and fear that you feel is part of the lesson you yourself have created. When you stop resisting the feeling and realize that the persons involved in the situations are just actors on the stage, then you are free to receive insights into what is going on.

Making Life Easy on Yourself

If you know yourself, then your life works. You do not have problems in one-to-one relationships. You do not set yourself up to be rejected or dumped on, lied to or ripped off. You do not set yourself up to be bored or frustrated, for you are in tune with and following your creative life path.

Remember that no one is going to take you by the hand and lead you step by step along the way. If you want insight, ask and you will receive. But you must make your own choices and decisions. It is your life. You are the writer, producer, and director, and you are playing all the roles. Create whatever you want. You have total freedom. It is only your thoughts that limit you.

Your dream symbols help you look at the very thought patterns that are governing your life. Dreams take you to a higher level of consciousness and understanding which has the power to transform your life and your world.

The whole purpose is to see objectively the life situations you are creating, survey the limitations and obstacles imposed through your own beliefs, and understand how best to work around or eliminate them. As you work on your own growth, all others will benefit; they will see your light, your knowledge and your truth.

PART II

Dream Symbol
Dictionary

ABANDONED   To abandon or leave behind characteristics or A
attitudes no longer needed for self-growth, or feeling of loss or
bewilderment because of giving away self-power to others;
abandonment of own inner resources and strength through
disregard. Need to work on loving, accepting yourself and taking responsibility for life direction.

ABDOMEN   Often represents solar plexus or third chakra: a
feeling of well-being and health indicates balanced emotions
and the centering of power or the life force; a feeling of pain
or distress means too much worry and tension. May also suggest how well you are able to digest life's experiences, taking
what is valuable, the positive lessons for growth, and discard-
ing the rest.

ABORIGINAL   The primitive or basic instinctive nature, unconscious or intuitional side of self. A part of self that is foreign to you, not known or understood, that is coming into
awareness.

ABORTION   Blocking a new birth or life direction within the
self. May be positive or negative ideas, projects, opportunities
or relationships; so examine carefully what is being cut off
from your experience.

ABOVE   Symbol above you suggests lift your sights, embrace
a new goal, draw upon third eye energy to tap higher creative
self. If something dark or ominous is hovering above, you are
weighing yourself down with unexamined fears or those you
have blown out of proportion.

ABSCESS   See *Boil.*

ABSORB   Merger or blending of separate elements; stronger
force, or aspect of self, taking over a less developed aspect.
Giving up free will, becoming absorbed, in cult, group or
something other than your own life path.

ABYSS   Confronting your own emptiness; you have cleaned
out the negative but now need to put the positive direction in
its place. Also, entering the unconscious to draw upon its

power. Facing a fear you have run away from in the past; there is no time like now.

ACCIDENT   Not paying enough attention to all parts of self, not integrating experiences; preoccupation. Going too fast; need to slow down, concentrate energy.

ACCOUNTANT   Detached self taking charge of its thoughts, words and actions. Balancing, giving and receiving energy.

ACE   Talent or ability which will carry you through in the game of life, as an ace up your sleeve. Also, 1 or 11. See *Numbers.*

ACID   Thoughts which have the power to corrupt or corrode. An acid test determines quality or real value of lessons learned; evaluation.

ACORN   Seed of great potential within self. A reminder to nurture and develop spiritual nature so that your full power and creative expression is realized.

ACTOR   Role you play, how others see you; a role you are playing at the moment which is serving some particular purpose. We all are actors; roles and life experiences are illusion. Our presentation of self changes as we grow; our roles change with expanding awareness and self-knowledge.

ADDICT   Giving up personal power, surrendering self-awareness to something or someone. Driven by fear and insecurity rather than self-responsibility, denying your own God-self or teacher within.

ADOLESCENT   Time of puberty; changes in physical and sexual awareness due to heightened kundalini power. Emotional growth goes more slowly. General confusion because of rapid changes and increased energy in the body; emotions and judgment are thrown off. To dream you are an adolescent when beyond those years may mean you are behaving like an adolescent, using poor judgment, going up and down emotionally; also, may mean a need for awakening and integrating sexual awareness. (The kundalini power kicks up again with great force at the time of menopause for both men and women.)

ADOPTION   Bringing in a brand new aspect of self, new beginning can be had now. You've earned it.

ADRIFT   Lack of goals, direction, purpose. Emotional self needs anchoring, loving and setting on course. Meditate to build energy, determine direction and accept self-responsibility.

ADULT   Mature self, viewing life from experience and greater sensitivity to self and others.

ADULTERY   Giving energy and attention to something that is separating self from inner growth; looking for outer pacifiers rather than resolving inner problems. Quality you are drawn to in another is blocked within yourself, or missing from your partnership. Also, may represent a merger and integration of male or female parts of self, depending upon sex of your dream partner. See *Sexual Intercourse*.

ADVERTISEMENT   Pay attention. Higher self or guidance is sending you a message.

AFFAIR   See *Adultery, Sexual Intercourse*.

AGREEMENT   Harmony within self or with another; a commitment. Promise or pact determining self-direction; may be positive or negative so understand nature of agreement and explore possible outcomes.

AIDS   See *Cancer*.

AIR CONDITIONER   Time for a cooling off period in your life.

AIR FORCE   Need for self discipline in your creative and spiritual practice. See *Military*.

AIRPLANE   Any flying aircraft indicates spiritual awakening, soaring to new heights. Note whether plane is on the ground, up in the air, taking off or landing; position reflects your spiritual awareness or perception concerning a particular problem or situation.

AIRPORT   Point of departure for spiritual awakening. See *Airplane*.

ALADDIN   Mystical part of self which transmutes energy, creates miracles; creative unconscious which is at your service once you learn how to use it.

ALARM   Caution or warning; you are veering off your path, approaching a questionable situation or relationship. Be aware and take responsibility for what needs to be changed.

ALBUM   Looking through a picture album means you are meeting the same lessons again in a new setting. Also, remembering past insights for use in the present. Source of pleasure; record of life experiences.

ALCHEMIST   Liberator from false concepts through transformation of awareness; higher self. See *Guru.*

ALCOHOL   Any alcoholic substance has a numbing effect, dulls the mind and feelings. May suggest hypersensitivity; a need for relaxation, meditation and raising the energy field to maintain inner balance. A need to open up and verbalize without feeling intimidated. Also, symbol of transformation, as Jesus turned water into wine; in this sense the transformation of consciousness to receive higher spiritual awareness.

ALIEN   A part of self we have ignored, rejected or misunderstood; a fear we have avoided. See *Foreign.*

ALIMONY   Retribution or karma. Paying off past actions, commitments or agreements you no longer choose to incorporate in your life.

ALLERGY   Extreme sensitivity due to physical constitution or emotional suppression.

ALLEY   A short cut to change directions; a redirection of plans. The way is narrow, limited, and must be followed closely. If dark represents an unknown and unfamiliar route.

ALLIGATOR   Tremendous power for verbal expression, which must be watched carefully so not used destructively. Fear of the misuse of verbal power. Integration of physical and emotional energy in a precarious balance.

ALPHABET   Basic symbols to communicate ideas and feelings; cultural interpretations of reality. Putting together concepts and feelings, but state of understanding still primitive. Individual letters may be interpreted through numerological significance. For example A, J, and S each = 1.

See chart below: also see *Numbers*.

1	2	3	4	5	6	7	8	9
A	B	C	D	E	F	G	H	I
J	K	L	M	N	O	P	Q	R
S	T	U	V	W	X	Y	Z	

ALTAR   Place of worship honoring source of life; commitment within the self. A sacrificing of the old and opening to the new; awareness of spiritual nature or God within.

AMBASSADOR   Guidance, a teacher; part of self you may call upon immediately to help resolve a problem, give insight.

AMBULANCE   An emergency; stop, pay attention to the situation at hand.

AMMUNITION   Use of power to protect or to destroy; positive or negative. Words may be ammunition to plead a cause; bullets may be ammunition for violence. Examine whether you are gathering resources for positive action, or planning to use thoughts, words and deeds to attack yourself or another.

AMPUTATION   To give up power, abilities, represented by removed limb or part. Cutting off unnecessary parts of self, which should be integrated, not rejected. For example, loss of right arm means you no longer are giving to self or others; left arm means no longer receiving energy needed to renew and rebuild. See individual body parts and *Body*.

AMULET   See *Charm*.

AMUSEMENT PARK   Relax, take a break from your serious attitudes toward living; laugh, have fun, loosen up. A merry-go-round or other circular ride by itself, however, suggests you are going around in circles, and need to get off, chart a new direction.

ANALYST   A need for self-exploration, to look within and make new discoveries. Be kind but honest with yourself; clean out negative, limiting concepts and open to higher levels of self-perception.

ANCHOR   Your lifeline, control point; freedom to choose emotional response and experience, ability to anchor self or to move ahead. If you have dropped anchor you are in control of emotions and are stopping to assimilate or sort out your life direction before moving on. If you have no anchor you drift from shore to shore without purpose and freedom to choose. But, anchors are temporary and should not be used to hold you back from venturing into new experiences and lessons.

ANCIENT   Truths that withstand the tests of time; timeless part of self that evolves through many lifetimes and lessons. Something old may indicate wisdom, empowerment; or parts of self no longer needed.

ANESTHESIA   Asleep at your control center; numbing of feelings, emotions; inability to see and hear with clarity. Avoidance of looking at your life and taking responsibility for self. Anesthesia does wear off, but you can hasten the process through meditation.

ANGEL   Messenger of God, highest ideal of spiritual self. Important dream message; listen!

ANGER   Frustration, hurt, disappointment in self because of unexpressed emotions and needs. You are always angry at yourself even though yelling at others. Insecurity, fear and negative programs are projected on others because of refusal to acknowledge that source of problem lies within. Anger may be used positively or negatively: to see areas for work on self, or to avoid responsibility and blame someone else.

ANIMAL   Instinctive part of self attuned to nature and survival, associated with second and third chakras. Also, the characteristics a specific animal represents to you, such as speed, cunning, power or wisdom. See individual animals.

ANKH   Spiritual power, emblem of life from ancient Egypt. Drawing upon ancient sources of knowledge.

ANKLE   Important to insure locomotion, movement; flexibility and support. See *Body.*

ANOREXIA   Depriving self of spiritual, emotional or physical nourishment; lack of self-love and acceptance. Striving for the attainment of an idealized ego-self which is empty and meaningless. Self-punishment.

ANT   Capable of carrying more than own weight; industrious, busy. Depending upon context, may be an annoyance, as letting little things bug you. Also, loss of individuality to a cause.

ANTENNA   Ability to transmit and receive energy. Your energy level determines what thoughts you are able to send and receive; you are always in communication on some level with the world around you. Examine what the antenna look like: long, short, bent, broken, to get an idea of your present capacity for attunement. Meditation builds strong antenna for enhanced control and finer tuning; you can learn to tune in or tune out and receive information from expanded states of consciousness.

ANTIDOTE   Corrects a wrong or imbalance; soothes and heals.

ANTIQUE   Usually represents old pattern, belief system or program which has served its purpose in your learning and growth and now should be released; afraid to change. A root to your past.

ANTISEPTIC   Cleanses and heals; protects against unwanted negative thoughts.

ANTLERS   Protection, assertiveness; powerful masculine part of self; a gift from your masculine self.

ANUS   Way to expel or rid yourself of thoughts and experiences no longer needed. Need for inner cleansing. Also, point of hidden stress which is difficult to feel; calls for release of tension and worry.

APE   Instinctual or primitive power, sexuality and strength; amusing antics, mimicking others rather than being yourself. See *Animal.*

APOSTLE   Higher self or teacher; follower of light and truth. Source for guidance and insight, rapid learning and problem solving. Pay attention.

APPLAUSE   Pat on the head from guidance; self-appreciation for a job well-done, whether great or small. Enhancing self-esteem or the need to do so.

APPLE   Healthful influence; new understanding, greater knowledge and wisdom. Energy and self-direction. Whether apple is ripe, beautiful, rotten or wormy suggests whether you are opening to new energy and insight, or need to clean out negativity and decay.

AQUARIUM   An emotional calming that's necessary now in your life. Showing you emotions in a relaxed and restful way. See *Fish, Water.*

ARCH   Support, frame. If spanning a window or passageway, suggests new opportunity or direction.

ARCHER   Setting your course or direction. Causal energy. See *Arrow* and *Bow.*

ARCHITECT   You are the architect and builder of your life; may mean planning a new direction, making blueprints for expansion and opportunity. Self-responsibility time.

ARCTIC   Frozen emotions, fear of opening up. Refusal to see that your true nature is flexible and pliable. Time to come out of cold storage and thaw.

ARENA   See *Stadium.*

ARGUMENT   Struggling with parts of self: paradoxes, conflicts, confusion. Mental self arguing with intuitive self. Holding on to old thought patterns which must be let go in order to move ahead, insure harmonious inner growth. Resolution comes from centering within, meditating, and drawing from a higher level of consciousness and understanding.

ARK   Noah's ark represents a balance of masculine and feminine energies in the emotional waters of life; emotional balance in partnerships. See *Boat.*

ARM   Expression of power or energy, extension of self. If right arm, sending or giving out; if left arm, receiving or bringing in. Depending upon dream context, arms may symbolize support, creativity or way of expressing yourself in the world. See *Body.*

ARMY   Need for physical self discipline in getting grounded. See *Military* and *War.*

ARRESTED   Loss of freedom; prevented from moving ahead. Take responsibility for actions and attitudes which have created the particular situation; change them into positive new understanding.

ARROW   Aspiration; energy directed toward a goal. A straight course for swift and easy accomplishment.

ART   Unconscious potential, abilities. Creative expression through relationships, music, writing, painting, or any art form. The art of living; how you are expressing yourself. Develop and experience more fully the creative self.

ARTHRITIS   Suppression; immobilizing self through rigid attitudes and beliefs. Lack of verbalization of feelings and needs. Self-punishment.

ASCETIC   Self-denial; efforts to grow inwardly by renouncing the outer world. Spiritual search, often misdirected through self-hatred and a poor self-image rather than the love of God. Cleansing, purification.

ASHES   Residue, essence, of spiritual purification by fire or light of God. Cleansing of body, mind and spirit, freeing self to move to new heights of understanding.

ASSEMBLY   See *Group*.

ASTHMA   Lack of protection of heart center, picking up too much stress and tension from those around you. Labored breathing results from an emotional overload. Relaxation, meditation are indicated to build and center energy.

ASTROLOGY   Relationship of planetary cosmic cycles to your own life; cosmic influence, energies. Guideline, map of aspects or constructs you may use to enhance learning and growth. Astrological configurations are stepping stones to higher awareness; you always have free will to determine how you will use, respond to, any influence on any level of your being. See *Horoscope*.

ASTRONAUT   Spiritual adventurer or explorer. Readiness to open to new awareness. No limitations.

ATHLETE   Integration of mental, physical and spiritual strengths through concentration and direction of energy. Strengthening qualities suggested by body parts being exercised (arms, head, back: see individual body parts); developing abilities suggested by equipment used (balance, flexibility, stamina). Need for enhancing awareness and building energy in the physical self.

ATOMIC BOMB   Enormous energy potential and responsibility for its creative use. May indicate great emotional suppression on the verge of exploding; verbalize, seek help, pay attention to own needs and take immediate action. Also, the awakening of kundalini fire or energy within, which is like an explosion into higher awareness.

ATTIC   Higher or spiritual self and what is going on in spiritual growth and development. Direction and insight determined by other symbols in the attic and the feelings you experience.

ATTORNEY   Advisor of universal laws; guidance. Acknowledge and understand differences in universal and human laws.

AUCTION   Freeing yourself of unwanted thoughts, things and experiences. An auction by choice means you have benefited from the past and are moving on; an auction by force means you are resisting change, harboring old ideas and resentments. Buying auctioned goods may be positive or negative, depending upon their quality and desirability.

AUDIENCE   Opportunity to express yourself and be heard; diverse parts of self are receptive to integration and direction, so goals may be formulated and new adventures begun. If audience is not listening, parts of yourself are unwilling to hear and respond to needed changes. You have to get their attention through self-love and acceptance.

AUDITION   Self-confidence, willingness to test yourself and see what you have learned. Trying out for a new part; opening the self to new experiences and roles.

AUDITORIUM   See *Building*.

AUNT   Feminine part of self; qualities or characteristics you identify with particular individual are projected aspects of yourself. See *Female*.

AURA   Energy field or light around you, charisma; strength or intensity reflects how easy or difficult you are making your life. The higher the energy, the more clarity you have. Meditation heightens and maintains the energy field.

AUTHOR   You are the writer of your life script. You can make it easy or difficult.

AUTOGRAPH   Identifying self. Look up name under *Alphabet* and *Numbers*.

AUTUMN   See *Season*.

AVALANCHE   Breaking loose of frozen emotions with a mighty jolt; opportunity to make changes before the freeze sets in again. Rejected parts of emotional self temporarily breaking free. See *Disaster*.

AVATAR   See *Guidance, Guru* and *Teacher*.

AWAKE   To dream you are awake, and aware that you are dreaming, is gaining a higher level of control over the dream state. New insight, awareness. See *Dream*.

AWARD   Something you've earned; insight, growth, ability. You have done well, so pause and appreciate yourself. Praise yourself for a good job.

AX   Tool for expressing power, creatively or destructively; such as, cutting away the old no longer needed, or destroying life possibilities. If someone is chasing you with an ax or vice versa, you are misusing power and are fearful of consequences. Redirect energy into positive and creative self-expression.

BABY   New birth within self; new aspects coming into being, new beginning. Openness, untapped potential for growth.   B

BABY-SITTING   Pay more attention to your inner child. Nurture and care for it.

BACK   The human back houses the spinal column, conductor of kundalini power of life force; whether back is straight, bent, weak or strong means how you are channeling the spiritual power in your everyday life. Strength of character or attitude in particular situation: spineless, broken, strong. Also, something now behind you in life; a part of self you have turned your back on. May mean backing up.

BADGE   Award for accomplishment, recognition or honor. Self-identity, status, how you see yourself.

BAG (Grocery)   Tools for nurturing self.

BAGGAGE   Unnecessary trips, programs or thought forms you carry around to define who you are; excess trivia and clutter. Often humorously presented, baggage means making something difficult that is really quite easy.

BAIT   Enticement, opportunity. A lure in a certain direction. Look and evaluate. Means pay attention.

BAKER   Alchemist; creative self. See *Cook*.

BALCONY   Higher level of perception; raising of consciousness. May mean you are on your way up. See *House*.

BALD   Unadorned, undisguised; symbolic of exposing crown chakra to higher learner and truth, dedication of self to spiritual growth. Loss of hair also represents loss of power. See *Hair*.

BALL   Completeness, wholeness; integration of conscious and unconscious, body, mind and spirit. If playing with a ball, a need for play and opening childlike awareness. If you throw the ball to someone, it is now the other's move; if you are catching or receiving, it is time for action—the ball is in your court.

BALLERINA   Balancing, joyful, uplifting. See *Dance*.

BALLOON   Uplifting of spirit, lighthearted, unrestricted. A popped balloon is the bursting of an illusion or fantasy, which gives momentary concern but lasting understanding. Riding in and controlling a balloon means soaring to new heights; drifting means you have no control and are at the mercy of the winds of change. Set your course.

BALLOT   Decision or judgment on matter at hand.

BAND   See *Music*.

BAND-AID   Trying to cover up poisons coming from within. Don't cover them up. Let the poisons come out so you can be healed.

BANK   Cosmic exchange, energy vault, unlimited resource. Collective unconscious; reservoir of all knowledge and ideas you may draw upon at any time. You make investments in yourself, deposits of talents and insights which will always be there; you are free to use the whole collective reserve to create whatever you want. Meditation enables you to tap these energies.

BANNER   See *Flag*.

BANQUET   Feast, celebration. You can create anything you choose. See *Food*.

BAPTISM   Spiritual awakening; rebirth into higher consciousness through Christ or Holy Spirit; death of limited thought patterns through awareness of God-self within. True baptism has nothing to do with ceremony or ritual, but is a sense of spiritual connection within the individual. This awakening allows you to see and understand the truth of your being, to know that all things are possible.

BAR, BAR ROOM   Usually represents looking for strength from without instead of within; need for self-acceptance, companionship, overcoming fear of rejection. Escape; numbing feelings and attunement to self and others. Also, transformation of consciousness, drinking of higher power. See *Alcohol*.

BARBER   Aspect of self concerned with image, power and strength. See *Hair*.

BARN   The need for protection and nurturing. See *Farm*.

BAROMETER   Indicator of your emotional climate, fluctuations and changes.

BARRICADE   Problem to be worked through before going on; a standstill until you resolve your dilemma. Self-imposed barrier to growth. See what it is and find the creative solution within.

BASEMENT   If you are in the basement or cellar of a house or building, you are working with sexual energy, understanding your sexual awareness and expression. People, objects and experiences reflect your use of sexual energy, degree of openness or suppression.

BASKET   Programs, ideas, and beliefs you're holding onto.

BATH   Purification, cleansing; also, time for relaxation and a little self-indulgence. See *Water*.

BATTERY   Life force or energy, connection to God-self. Regular recharge through meditation keeps your battery high: no energy, no insight.

BATTLE   See *War.*

BEACH   Borderline or bridge between conscious and unconscious; standing on beach enables you to pull tremendous energy from the ocean, using the power of the unconscious to center you and actualize life goals. Sand is healing, grounding energy. If thrown on the beach by a wave or fish, you now have time to regroup and build energy after going through an emotional period. If stranded on a deserted shore, you have cut yourself off from your wealth of unconscious resources. Go within and you will find the solution you seek.

BEADS   Need for inner focusing. See *Art.*

BEAR   Strength, power; inconsistent emotional energy, not to be trusted: can be violent or cuddly, charming or crabby. See *Animal.*

BEARD   Strength, wisdom, masculinity. See *Hair.*

BEAUTY SHOP   Lift up your self esteem. Create a better self image.

BEAVER   Working hard to dam up emotional self, stop emotional currents from opening and flowing. Hiding from resolving emotional problems. See *Animal.*

BED   Bridge between conscious and unconscious; a return to the universal womb or power source. Beds play important roles in our lives: rest, relaxation, rejuvenation, nurturing, sexual intimacy. Desire for safety, awareness of Divine protection. Special relationship with many levels of self; expression of individuality: you make your own bed or life experiences.

BEDSPREAD   See *Cover.*

BEE   Wonderful, integrative force; kinship with nature; maker of sweetness in life. Also, stinging thoughts and remarks, gossip; confusion of activity, letting little things bug you.

BEER   See *Alcohol.*

BEETLE   Scarab beetle represents eternal life, spiritual awakening, as used in ancient Egypt and other cultures.

BELL   Attunement, awakening to new insight, centering and harmonizing with Divine consciousness. Signal to be alert, sensitive to present and forthcoming experiences, or to dream message.

BELT   Holding things together, insuring smooth operation, as a belt on machinery. When around waist, may represent stress and tension in third chakra or solar plexus; stomach tied up.

BENCH   Place for rest and relaxation, take time out. See *Chair*.

BIBLE   Spiritual study; humankind's search for enlightenment. The closest document to truth, but must be interpreted symbolically.

BICYCLE   Need for balance in your life. Balance energies before moving ahead under full steam.

BIG   Anything big usually denotes the size of one's mental and emotional investment in the symbol or what it represents. Out of proportion in importance or value; making a mountain out of a molehill. Also, the potential of an idea, plan, or oneself; a big house or a large vehicle means great potential and power.

BILL   Karmic repayment, depending upon whether sending or receiving.

BILLIARDS   As in all games, suggests competition, skill, concentration, winning and losing. See *Game*.

BINOCULARS   Ability to see with clarity.

BIRD   Spiritual freedom; ability to soar to higher awareness. Freedom from material ties.

BIRTH CONTROL   See *Contraceptive, Birth*.

BIRTH   Opening a new direction, new possibilities. See *Baby*.

BIRTHDAY   Celebration of new part of yourself coming into being. A new birth.

BITE   Sink your teeth into the problem or lesson. See *Chew*.

BLACK   Unconscious, unknown parts of self, sometimes those we have rejected through fear. See *Color*.

BLACKSMITH   Forging strong new forms; strength, power, masculinity.

BLANKET   See *Cover.*

BLESS, BLESSING   Divine protection, given as a gift of love. Form of initiation; self-acceptance or recognition of progress in growth and understanding.

BLIND   Need to develop inner spiritual vision; you see but do not see. You are not making the right choices, blinding yourself to truth. Look within and try again.

BLISTER   Eruption of emotions, poisonous thoughts and feelings. If still in blister form, you need to release disharmony in order to heal. See *Boil.*

BLIZZARD   Going through a chilling emotional upheaval and being unwilling to look at tremendous changes and possibilities for growth. A heavy snow job on self or another; examine motives. See *Snow, Avalanche.*

BLOOD   Life force or energy. If you are bleeding you are losing energy; someone is taking your energy, or you are draining yourself through worry, fear or lack of balance. See what area of body is bleeding. See *body parts* and *Chakra.*

BLOSSOM   A job well done; you have sown and reaped beauty, a beautiful expression of self. See *Flower, Bouquet.*

BLUE   Spirituality, relaxation, happiness. Depending upon context, may mean sadness or disappointment, as when feeling blue; frozen emotions, as when one turns blue with cold; or hurting and bruised from experiences.

BOAT   Your emotional self. If at the helm you are in control; if your boat is drifting, you are not in charge of your emotional life. If sinking you are allowing your emotions to pull you under, so take a good look at what is pulling you down in day to day living. Through self-examination, making positive choices, you can change negative emotional trips.

BODY   Your temple, earth suit, expression of self in a space-time world. A masculine or feminine body represents that particular side of yourself; child's body is playful, intuitive side of self. Vehicle for learning lessons while on the earth plane, so important to keep the body healthy and strong. See different body parts.

BOIL   Poisons erupting from within. Suppressed emotions coming out in unhealthy directions. See *Blister*. Boiling water or other liquid is getting things moving, purifying, cleansing. If pot is boiling over means too much negative energy, high emotions, anger; out of balance.

BOMB   See *Atomic Bomb*.

BONE   Foundation, belief systems, strength or support. Essential for proper functioning of all other parts.

BOOK   Your book of life, or what your purpose is in this lifetime. Knowledge of life plan. Pay attention; important lessons coming up.

BOOKKEEPER   See *Accountant*.

BOSS   The critic within self, which can be a creative or destructive influence. Guidance giving you helpful instructions. The nature of the relationship with your own boss.

BOTTLE   Capped bottle means closed or locked up inside, but can easily break through to new awareness. Old empty bottle is discarded part of self you do not need anymore. If you receive a message from floating bottle, one washed up by the sea, the unconscious self is offering an answer to a problem.

BOUQUET   Celebration of growth. Pat yourself on the back you've done well. Also see *Flower, Blossom*.

BOW (Archer's)   Power to set goals, force to accomplish them. Flexibility. Strength which can aim the arrow of achievement. See *Archer, Arrow*.

BOW   To honor the God within; to recognize and honor a part of self.

BOWEL   Deep or hidden feelings; guts of a situation, basic understanding. Process of cleansing and releasing the past, unused and unneeded experiences and ideas.

BOWL   Vessel for nurturing self. See *Cup*.

BOX   The games you set up, little realities you create, limits you impose upon yourself. One endeavors continuously to break out of boxes and expand vision.

BOY   Masculine child part of self; growing masculine qualities within. Physical, outer expression which is open and vulnerable.

BRACELET   See *Jewelry, Hand.*

BRACES   Need to verbalize with love. Correct your manner of speech.

BRAID   Spiritual strength; unity; interweaving of body, mind and spirit. See *Rope.*

BRAIN   Cosmic computer or storage bank. Although associated with the rational mind, the brain transmits information from both conscious and unconscious, transcending the third dimension of time-space. Expand awareness of own power and opportunity; develop interdimensional understanding of self and others. Brain power lies dormant; meditation awakens it.

BRAKE   Control point. Caution, use brakes when needed and slow down; no brakes means out of control, danger. Stop, examine a particular situation before moving ahead; slow down before moving on.

BRANCH   See *Limb.*

BRASS   The inner self that can be tarnished unless it's polished and buffed to shine forth its light.

BREAD   Fellowship; communion with others in awareness that we are all a part of God's body. Body as the temple of God; process of learning life's lessons through staff of life or God awareness. Meditation or communion with God is the bread of life, the realization of our oneness with all things.

BREAK   To break something is to make a change, dispel illusion. Also, pushing too hard and need to slow down; lack of awareness.

BREAST FEED   Feeding emotional support to yourself or others. Protect your own energy and watch that you give to others only what you can afford to give away. See *Nursing.*

BREAST   Heart chakra, God or love center within. Nurturing, comfort, unconditional love.

BREATH   Life force, kundalini. Breath regulates bodily functions and consciousness: slow breathing means centering, relaxing bodymind energy; fast strong breathing suggests acceleration of power. If you are out of breath, you are out of balance, going too fast; slow down and reorganize.

BRICK   Strength, endurance. Building a new direction, remodeling.

BRIDE, BRIDEGROOM   When both bride and bridegroom are in a dream, they represent the merger of masculine and feminine qualities within the self; a new beginning with maturity and more responsibility. Marriage is union of body, mind and spirit. Bride is new beginning with higher awareness of feminine self; bridegroom is new beginning with higher awareness of masculine self.

BRIDGE   A transition, leaving the old and entering the new. A new opportunity for growth; threshold of a new direction in life. It may represent bridging levels of consciousness, the creative-intuitve with the intellectual.

BRIEFCASE   Parts of your self identity and programs that you're carrying around with you.

BRONZE   Strength, progress, ingenuity; protective, strengthening covering. Earlier lessons learned in your development.

BROOK   Gentle emotional expression; spiritual healing. Problems, concerns are easy to overcome, resolve by own effort.

BROOM   Clean up your act. Get your house in order and make way for the new.

BROTHER   Masculine part of self. Qualities in self you project on brother or brother figure. Perception of relationship with actual brother or person brother represents.

BROWN   Earthiness; grounding. Get back in touch with physical side of self; too much emphasis on mental and spiritual; you are out of balance.

BRUSH (Hair)   To untangle ourselves from problems which cost us energy. Organizing energy. Can also be used to mean to set things aside. You're brushing things aside.

BUBBLE   See *Balloon.*

BUD   Getting ready to open to new opportunities; be patient.

BUDDHA   Master teacher; higher spiritual self; source of spiritual energy and truth.

BUFFALO   Ancient strength. To intimidate, puzzle, mystify.

BUG   Little things are bugging you; little annoyances. Get your energy up and you will have a better perspective.

BUILD, BUILDING   To build is to create something new; expanding or enhancing a part of your life. A large building is a tremendous energy source; suggests you have great opportunities, tremendous potential and a big destiny to fulfill.

BULB   Light bulb is an idea when lit; if dark, meditate to expand energy field, get new ideas. A flower bulb represents potential for growth and unfoldment; time for planting.

BULL   Strong; stubborn, bull-headed. Masculine aggressiveness.

BULLDOZER   Great power to build up or tear down. May mean clear away the old, get ready for the new. Get rid of old ideas. Depending upon dream context, may mean destruction of limits, construction of new foundations, or both.

BURGLAR   Something is robbing the self of energy, wasting the life force; often is your inability to say "no" to demands made upon your time and thought. Negativity, fear, anxiety, guilt and resistance are examples of inner robbers.

BURIAL   Death of old emotions and attitudes no longer needed for your highest growth. Death of fear and insecurity. Also, hiding from life, burying aliveness, emotions and sensitivity. See *Death.*

BURN   Purification, cleansing. See *Fire.*

BUS   Tremendous potential for self expression. See *Vehicle.*

BUSINESS   All parts of ourselves working together to bring forth the results that we chose to accomplish.

BUSINESS PERSON   The organizational part of self.

BUTCHER   Aggression, anger; chopping up the self into parts, rather than integrating, achieving wholeness. Fear, insensitivity.

BUTTER   Sweetness, nurturing; slippery, greasy. Also, false flattery, as buttering up someone or yourself.

BUTTERFLY   Rebirth in higher form; transmutation of energy. The beauty that comes from trusting the process of growth through all its ups and downs, emerging triumphant in new awareness.

BUTTOCKS   Stop, sit down and face the problem.

BUTTON   Used humorously, need to button your lip (close your mouth). If unbuttoning, you are opening up. Can also mean someone is pushing your button to see if you will react.

BUY   See *Shop*.

BUZZARD   Constructive symbol meaning to clean up and clear out old decaying attitudes and ideas. Be willing to release and let go of those ideas and relationships no longer beneficial for your growth. It is all part of the natural process of things.

CABIN   Rest and relaxation is needed.

C

CABINET   See *Drawer*.

CABLE   Communication with others and with self. Represents level and degree of openness to send and receive messages; a strong connection. As wire, suggests strength and durability. See *Wire*.

CACTUS   Caution; look but do not touch. Apparent beauty may have painful repercussions. Negative part of self that grew without much care or nurturing, and may hurt self or others through lack of awareness. A prickly problem. Gossip, pointed remarks, sticking it to yourself or someone.

CAFE   See *Restaurant*.

CAGE   Self-created prison; fear of being trapped by your own limitations. Fear of self-expression. Cage door is never locked; you are free to leave through the doorway to freedom, your own awareness.

CAKE   Celebration and nurturing. Luxurious treat, special gift.

CALCULATOR   Self-evaluation; adding things up. Depending on context, may indicate a harsh, judgmental self; a need for balancing energy flow. Also, figuring out a situation.

CALENDAR   Time or the timing of a project; unfoldment. Seasonal growth. See *Time* and *Season*.

CALF   Youthfulness, gaiety, playfulness. Killing the fatted calf indicates abundance, celebration. The calf of your leg represents strength, flexibility, movement.

CAMCORDER   See *Movie.*

CAMEL   Endurance; inner resources to draw upon when making life's journey. Perseverance in the face of difficulties to be resolved.

CAMERA   Perception of experiences; record of life to draw upon for learning. Learn to see the positive lesson for growth in every life picture or experience, and your photo album will be filled with the essence of joy and love.

CAMOUFLAGE   Hiding one's true self.

CAMP   To camp in nature is to reestablish contact with the earth, develop a sense of grounding; to commune with self and life in an uncluttered, basic way. To harmonize with nature, tap into a deeper, stronger energy source. If military camp, see *Military* and *War.*

CAN   If unopened, part of self is sealed off. Rusty tin can represents old beliefs, attitudes no longer needed. Also artificial, as in canned laughter. To dispel or rid the self of something, as in canning an old habit.

CANAL   Narrow emotional direction; emotional path which may save you time and energy, but has little room for variation.

CANCER   Anger, frustration, disappointment; fear eating away inside you. Lack of self-love; inability to look at inner disharmony or refusal to do so. Suppression of any kind is dangerous to physical, mental and emotional health; verbalize, get things up and out, be honest with yourself.

CANDLE   Light within. Each soul has a light, and ability to see with clarity depends upon the strength of the inner light. The true nature of your being is light. Awareness determines brightness.

CANDY   A treat, or can mean you need extra energy. Spoiling yourself through over indulgence instead of following a balanced plan for living.

CANE   Support, helpful influence. You may need assistance in some project or plan. Helpmate.

CANNIBAL   Depriving part of the self in order to strengthen another part; destroying parts of the self through insensitivity, hidden hungers, ignorance. Living off energies of others instead of generating own creative energy source. Need to awaken a wider spiritual knowledge to see the interconnection of all life.

CANOE   Maintaining emotional balance. See *Boat*.

CANTEEN   Tools that are easily carried to nurture the emotional self.

CANYON   Approaching unknown territory; the unconscious. Specific but limited lessons to be learned before venturing back out into the open; narrow pathway.

CAP   Cover or protection, point at which one opens, closes, or seals off. See *Hat*.

CAPSIZE   Trying to avoid situations you find uncomfortable; getting dumped emotionally. Fear of unconscious, emotional self; feelings of guilt, impotency. Get back in your boat and steer through the rough water.

CAPTAIN   Higher self who guides you through the emotional waters of life. If not at the helm, you are out of control and need to take responsibility for yourself.

CAPTIVE   Giving up your power to others, not being assertive. Holding resentment toward others for letting them walk on you. Forget the self-pity trip and take your power back; establish a responsible and creative life direction.

CAR   You in daily physical life. The larger the vehicle the more potential you are using to manifest what you want. If going up hill, you are going the right way. Down hill is the wrong direction. Both up and down, you are not in control and your energy is scattered. If you are not in the driver's seat, who are you letting drive your car? Get behind the wheel and take charge of your life and its direction. Note the color of the vehicle and how many people, if any, are with you. See *Number* and *Color*.

CARBURETOR   Blending together spiritually, emotionally and physically. Balance.

CARDS   Seeing life as a game, a gamble. Focusing on winning and losing instead of growing; competing instead of creating. If a fortune teller is reading your cards, reflects own psychic attunement; or seeking your destiny from outer, not inner sources. Remember that you create from within.

CARPENTER   Building your life. Repairs, maintenance, additions, subtractions; see what you are doing and what is needed.

CARPET   Grounding, insulation, protection. Luxury you may enjoy. Also, do not pull the rug out from under yourself; stay centered and positive

CARROT   Lure, appeal. See *Food.*

CASKET   See *Coffin.*

CASTLE   Reach for your dreams. You can create all your dreams and bring them into reality.

CASTRATE   To take away masculine power, assertiveness, strength; to destroy the ability to feel and create.

CAT   Feminine part of self. See *Animal.*

CATACOMB   Inner being; hidden aspects of self. Wandering through the depths of many lifetimes; integration.

CATERPILLAR   Limited knowledge; unaware of potential and beauty.

CATHEDRAL   See *Church.*

CAVE   Unconscious mind; unexplored parts of self. Great treasures lie within as you continue the adventure of self-discovery.

CEILING   Limit or protection. Eventually you outgrow protective coverings; understanding relationship between need for protection and need for expansion is important for continued well-being.

CELEBRATE   See *Party, Ceremony.*

CELEBRITY   Usually represents your teachers. Note if they are male (masculine power) or female (feminine power). If it's a comedian you need to use humor, become more lighthearted. Look name up under *Alphabet* and *Numbers*.

CELIBACY   Fear of intimacy. Misguided spiritual thinking that enlightenment precludes experiencing the sexual energy. Blocking off lower chakras or energy centers; energies within must be integrated, merged into a higher awareness. Retreating within self to know the self; awakening spiritual identity.

CENTAUR   Animal, instinctual, nature; functioning more from instinct than higher perception. If in a relationship suggests more a sexual orientation than genuine loving. Awareness of need to integrate higher and lower natures, physical and spiritual energy.

CEREMONY   Initiation, celebration or graduation.

CESSPOOL   All the negative programs, limiting ideas you are harboring. Time to clean up emotionally, releasing and forgiving self and others.

CHAIN   Strength; many links or parts working together. Also, a link by itself means isolation, weakness; or the key, as in the missing link. Restriction or limit, as you become chained to habits and ideas which hold you back from further growth and achievement.

CHAIR   Your attitudes, position in life; how you see yourself, identity. Also, comfort and centering, especially if a rocking chair; the rocking motion builds and centers energy.

CHAKRA   One of seven major energy centers in etheric body; energy transformer. May suggest opening or blocking of a particular center. Chakras include the root chakra, sexual chakra, solar plexus, heart chakra, throat chakra, third eye, and crown chakra.

CHALK   Means of self expression, look up color.

CHAMELEON   Adaptability; flexibility. Fickleness; constantly changing roles, whimsical.

CHAMPAGNE   See *Alcohol*.

CHANDELIER   Very elegant, beautiful reflection of your inner light.

CHARM   Effort to get in touch with spiritual power. Looking for answers without rather than within. Old wives' tales, belief systems, which may or may not have any validity. Divine protection comes from within. The rabbit's foot did not help the dead rabbit.

CHART   Blueprint for goals; plan for your life. See *Map*.

CHEAT   Trying to get away with something rather than being honest with yourself.

CHECK (Paycheck)   Paying off dues. Being rewarded for a job well done. See also *Salary*.

CHEF   See *Cook*.

CHESS   Game of life. The intricacies of competition, defeat and victory. There is an easier way to go.

CHEST   A place of stored or hidden treasure. Ideas, attitudes or belief systems that are not yet out in the open. If body; heart chakra, God or love center within.

CHEW   Breaking down, assimilating knowledge or information; thinking something over, sorting out, sifting through. Chewing nails or something too tough to swallow indicates a problem you are unwilling to handle, or is not yours in the first place; also, lack of verbalization.

CHICKEN   Usually presented humorously: may mean hen-pecked or giving away power. Fearful and flighty, lack of self-assurance; cowardly, not working through problems. See *Hen*. Also *Food*.

CHILDREN   Aspects of yourself, such as vulnerability, innocence, openness, flexibility, playfulness. Your own children mirror your attitudes and beliefs. Often suggests you have forgotten the child part of self.

CHIMNEY   Extension of self; channel for cleansing and releasing, as smoke goes up a chimney. See *House*.

CHOCOLATE   Giving oneself a treat for a job well done. Need for nurturing. See *Candy*.

CHOIR   Spiritual harmony; working with others in bringing about uplifting experiences; integrated, harmonious parts of self.

CHOKE   Blockage of kundalini power in throat or fifth chakra, usually through lack of verbalization. To choke on food is inability to digest or accept certain experiences, ideas.

CHRIST   God within you. Heart center or love energy within. Master teacher.

CHRISTMAS   Celebration, awakening of love power, spiritual birth, giving and receiving of higher awareness. A reflection of past ties with family and friends, meaning they imparted to your life; strengths you can draw upon in the present.

CHURCH   May represent an outer appearance of spirituality rather than an attunement within your own inner temple. Jesus never had a church, but taught among the people. Also, a worshipful consciousness within the self; a need to awaken awareness in acknowledgment of a Higher Power.

CIGAR, CIGARETTE   A pacifier, much like a thumb for a child. Something worthless except for the value you give it, such as, relaxation or calming nervous energy. A harmful influence that is not necessary. A worthless tool.

CIRCLE   Wholeness, completeness; no beginning and no end; infinity. The circle may mean you have completed a cycle or have grown into a wholeness of body, mind and spirit. If presented as a merry-go-round or movement in circles, you are not getting on with your life and lessons; you literally are going around in circles.

CIRCUMCISE   Cutting off and throwing away a vital part of yourself; to cut yourself off from your own power, sexuality, feelings or emotions.

CIRCUS   Recapture your childlike enjoyment of life. Also, your life is like a circus with too much going on, quantity but not quality. Learn to laugh at yourself, enjoy self and others.

CITY   Intense networking of people or parts of self; you are being forced to communicate and cooperate. A need for community and working together, reaching out to others. Intense energy, need for balance and taking time to smell the roses.

CLAM   Not communicating well, keeping everything inside. Verbalize more and express yourself.

CLAMP   Holding yourself together in the midst of stress and tension; protection.

CLASS   Learning a new lesson. Taking a particular course in life. See *School*.

CLAW   Jealousy, anger, or holding on too tightly to a situation.

CLAY   You are ready to mold yourself into something new, creating new realities in your life. A certain situation can be molded, reshaped, changed into harmonious experience.

CLEAN   Shining up old parts of self. To be made as new. See *Wash*.

CLIFF   A point in your life which calls for radical change. If you are pushed off or jump off a cliff, you are being instructed to make a decision, move ahead, and venture into unexplored territory. Falling off a cliff may also suggest being out of control; do not get yourself into something you cannot get out of.

CLIMB   If climbing upward you are going the right way. If climbing down you are going the wrong direction in life.

CLOCK   Time is of the essence; get on with your life. It all depends on timing. Note numbers on clock or what time it is. See *Numbers*.

CLOSET   A storage place for attitudes, ideas and memories. You probably need to clean out a few. Also, hiding or closing yourself off from the mainstream of living.

CLOTH   The materials with which you create your life. Note color.

CLOTHES   The roles or games you play, attitudes you have. A costume dream may suggest a past life experience, presented because the lessons you are going through now are the same ones you were confronted with then.

CLOTHESLINE   Used humorously, take a look at your "hangups." Clothes are roles you play. See *Clothes*.

CLOUD   A light, fluffy cloud is the rising of spiritual consciousness, inner peace. A dark cloud is low energy, depression; you are not looking at your lessons. An emotional downpour may be imminent.

CLOWN   Ability to laugh at oneself, see the humor in all situations. One learns more through laughter and lightness; laughter heals. Enjoy life, dare to be yourself.

COACH   A higher teacher is there to help you along. If a stage coach, it's a part of self used for display and fun.

COAL   Unknown energy sources within self; potential.

COAT   Warmth or protection; also, covering up or hiding emotions, not letting people see who you really are.

COBRA   Kundalini power (life force or creative energy) is rising up through the energy centers or chakras. Awakening to inner power. See *Snake*.

COBWEBS   Talents not used, ideas not put into practice. Abilities sitting undisturbed.

COCK   If crowing, warning or signal. Ego; aggressiveness, masculine nature.

COFFEE   Relaxation, stimulation, pacification; habit to examine; depends upon what coffee represents to you.

COFFIN   The ending of a situation or experience; closing off a part of self. Boxed in, no growth. Time to move out and get on with it. Can also mean "case closed." See *Burial*.

COIN   See *Money*.

COLD   If something feels cold or you feel cold, warm up emotions and feelings; do not cut yourself off from sensitivity to self and others.

COLLAPSE   An undermining of the physical, mental, emotional or spiritual self. Pay attention and repair, change, whatever is called for.

COLLEGE   An advanced course in learning and growth. See *School*.

COLOR   Rate of vibration, harmony within your energy field. The colors have different vibrations, properties, and represent different levels of awareness. You choose to wear colors that harmonize with your own energy field. Various colors are:
  Red – energy.
  Rose, pink – love.

Orange – energy, peace.

Yellow – peace.

Green – healing, growth.

Blue – spirituality.

Turquoise – healing, spirituality.

Indigo – spirituality, divine protection.

Violet, purple, lavender – wisdom, knowledge, divine
   protection.

Grey – fear.

Black – unknown, unconscious.

White – truth, purity.

Brown – grounding.

Gold – Christ light, divine consciousness.

Silver – spiritual protection, truth.

Some colors are also listed separately.

COMB   Untangling a situation. Still taking out tangles.

COMEDY   Do not take yourself so seriously. Remember everything is a set-up to help you learn your lessons. Lighten up;
laughter heals.

COMET   Powerful unleashing of energy which causes growth
among the populace. Heralding of self growth, tremendous
creative potential, great success; awakening of self and others.

COMMUNE   Moving away from the stream of society and
doing things your own way; working together with others
toward a common goal.

COMPASS   Stop and get your direction in life; if feeling lost,
tune in to inner sense, inner path, and you will find the way.
Direction you are now headed. See *North, South, East, West*.

COMPLEXION   Reflection of inner self; how you appear to
self and others, how you see yourself.

COMPUTER   Your mind is a computer. Your thoughts words
and actions create your reality. Watch what you program, this
will determine your life.

CONDOM   See *Contraceptive*.

CONDUCTOR   Higher self. Planning, leading, directing level
of awareness.

CONFESSION   Opening up, lightening one's burden, cleansing of emotional and mental negativity. The absolution of sins represents a recognition of attitudes and behaviors which are destructive to growth. Forgiving oneself is the key to fully living in the present. Need to verbalize, talk about concerns and share with others.

CONSTIPATION   Emotional suppression; holding on to ideas, attitudes and experiences no longer needed for balanced and healthful functioning.

CONSTRUCTION   You are in the process of rebuilding who and what you are.

CONTEST   Parts of yourself vying for some reward.

CONTRACEPTIVE   Preventive measure, used to protect health or to prevent new directions in the self from emerging. Barrier; cutting off creative power. Depends upon context of dream and feeling level, whether positive or negative influence.

CONVENT   Spiritual regrouping or retreat. A need to go within, explore the feminine self, and integrate experiences before venturing into new lessons. Hiding from self, growth, or calling in the world. Effort to discover the spiritual part of self without the understanding that comes from many and varied life experiences. Closing off of self from active integrative spiritual growth. See *Monastery*.

CONVENTION   A meeting of many parts of self. See *Group*.

CONVICT   See *Criminal*.

COOK   Putting together the many ingredients of your life; observe what, and how you are proceeding. If something is burning you are working under too much pressure. Cooking up mischief. Also, you are really cooking, getting on with it, filled with ideas and action.

COPPER   Conductor of heat, energy, life force; beauty, strength, flexibility, health.

CORAL   Beauty coming from the depths of the emotions.

CORK   Lightness of spirit; ability to rise above circumstances, emotional ups and downs. Versatility, flexibility.

CORNER   Convergence of energies, point of change for new direction. Having an edge or advantage in a situation, as a corner on the market. Being backed into a corner means it is now time to make a decision to free yourself from a limiting situation.

CORPSE   A part of the self that has died: feelings, attitudes, beliefs. May be positive or negative aspects. Usually suggests deadened feelings and responses; fear has closed you off from own aliveness. See *Death*.

COSMETICS   Enhancing the self-image to bolster confidence. Also, hiding from one's true self, not seeing inner beauty. If heavily made up you are not recognizing inner worth, demeaning yourself, focusing on outer rather than inner values.

COST   What are you willing to pay for your happiness and growth in life? It requires self discipline and self responsibility. See *Numbers*.

COTTON   Parts coming together in harmony.

COUCH   Used as a psychiatrist's couch, represents need to know oneself, to examine programs and beliefs on a deeper level. If a couch in your living room, symbolizes something that is going on in your daily life; notice color, size, shape.

COUNTRY   Images of the country or countryside suggest time for growth, creativity, relaxation; reattunement to childlike awareness of nature. Many creative choices or options.

COUPLE   Two parts of self. Note whether they're masculine or feminine.

COURT   Going to court or in a court room, you are judging yourself, perhaps being driven by hidden guilts and fears. The judge and jury represent your higher self, guidance, or critic. See *Judge, Jury*.

COURTYARD   Protected growth, not subjected to the winds of change. Growth we can readily realize and actualize. See Yard.

COVENANT   Pact with God or yourself. A commitment to self or another.

COVER   Depending upon context, a protection or a hiding from self and others.

COW   Often used as a sacred symbol, represents nurturing and feeding; sustenance through love. Motherhood.

COWARD   Afraid to see yourself as you actually are, to manifest goals, get on with growth. Fears are preventing you from daring to be yourself.

COWBOY, COWGIRL   One who loves the outdoors. Man or woman controlling their animal instincts, roping and corralling them; harnessing your power.

CRAB   Necessary to move ahead or problem solve in an indirect manner; or, you are now moving sideways rather than straight ahead. Your current disposition: crabby.

CRACK   Part of the wall you have built is opening; something in need of repair mentally, physically or emotionally. Depends upon whether crack suggests decay or breaking through.

CRADLE   Nurturing a new part of self; need for loving and nurturing.

CRASH   See *Wreck*.

CRATER   Old memory of explosive experience. An opening to the unconscious.

CRAYONS   Creating colorful expression. See *Art*.

CRAZY   One who refuses to accept responsibility for having chosen to live in this reality; one who acts out primal urges of man. Also, lightheartedness; acting on the spur of the moment without thinking.

CREAM   Richness, opportunity; nurturing. If lotion, protection for body.

CREDIT CARD   Getting something which you'll have to pay for at a later date. Nothing is free; you will have to earn it.

CREDIT   You have done something well and have a bonus coming. Agreement of responsibilities.

CREEK   If dry it means that nothing emotional is happening in your life now. If there's water, note the flow, gentle = harmonious; heavy = you're going through a lot.

CREST   As a coat of arms, one's sense of identity or roots. If the crest of a wave, an emotional turn around; or feeling on top of everything.

CRICKET   Good omen, good luck, prosperity. A helpful insight; your conscience or guidance. Also, a little thing is bugging you.

CRIMINAL   Cheating on oneself and limiting one's potential. Making own laws out of fear rather than following inner source of guidance and creative attunement.

CRITIC   Self-discipline; if used wrongly can block achievement of highest good for fear of censure and making a mistake. Humankind's limited awareness does not give one the wisdom to judge self or others.

CROOK   One who steals from and undermines self. See *Criminal.*

CROP   What you sow you reap. Represents growth that comes from self-love and nurturing. If a small crop in your fields, you have been negligent in using talents and abilities, short of self-appreciation and self-love.

CROSS   Originally the mystical symbol for man, meaning perfect balance. The point of intersection was centered, representing the heart chakra as opened with three chakras above and three below.

CROSSROAD   A choice in direction you soon will make. If you are shown a forked road, the right path is the way of intuition and creativity and the left path is the way of the intellect. (Hint: take the right.)

CROWD   Many parts of self. Dream context would show whether noisy, peaceful, purposeful, or whatever, indicating how well different parts of self are integrated.

CROWN   A crown of gold or jewels means praise; keep going, good work. It may symbolize an initiation into higher awareness. A crown of thorns means you are working on things, but there is still a lot to do; try to get out of your tendency to act the martyr and look at lessons more clearly.

CRUCIFIXION   Undeserving punishment of self. Lack of self-love results in need to bare one's soul, crucify the self. To "suffer for the Lord" is tragic programming; if you expect life to be difficult, it is. The only things to crucify or eliminate are negativity and limitation.

CRUISE   Emotional journey. It's a big vessel so it means you're really cruising emotionally through life, easy going!

CRUTCH   Temporary assistance, support, used when one feels unable to draw upon own inner strength and wisdom. Focusing on handicap rather than resolving the problem.

CRY   Release of stress and tension, frustrration; if tears of joy may be resolving a problem, working through blocks; or emotional release from appreciation of beauty, integration of life, filling up with wonderment.

CRYSTAL   Energy conductor and storehouse.

CUDDLE   Expression of love, caring, warmth and affection. Need for TLC.

CULT   Group of people or parts of self following belief systems without question. Cutting self off from opportunities by buying someone else's truth. One ultimately must move beyond systems: dare to be you.

CUP   Spiritual heart of self. If overflowing you are attuned to divine love; if empty you are walling self off from love energy, life force within.

CUPID   Growth in love relationships; taking a risk. Good and self-explanatory symbol.

CURSE   See *Hex*.

CURTAIN   Closed curtains mean to hide away, close off from self and others. Opened curtains mean opportunity for growth, seeing beyond present situation. If draped over something suggests you are hiding aspects of self.

CUT   Depending upon context, may mean cutting away old parts of self-beliefs, attitudes, programs no longer needed. If bleeding from a cut, you are losing energy. See *Scissors, Knife*.

DAGGER   See *Knife*.

DAM   Walled-off emotions; holding back from others. If dam has burst you are releasing stored up emotions. See *Beaver, Flood*.

D

DANCE　Lightheartedness, happiness, joy. The dance of life. Also, dancing around a problem instead of resolving it.

DANGER　Be alert, aware; feeling of impending change with no clarity. New aspects of self coming into being which are presently unfamiliar, hence fearful.

DARK　Something unknown emerging from the unconscious. Walking through a situation with low energy and little clarity. Meditate, get your energy up, and turn on the inner light.

DART　If throwing darts suggests pointed, harmful thoughts and words; stinging remarks. Also, aiming for a target or goal.

DAUGHTER　Feminine child part within self. Also, qualities you project on your own daughter; nature of relationship with daughter or person in that role.

DAWN　Beginning, new awakening, insight and understanding. Rising to the tasks before you.

DAY　Daytime suggests enough light or energy to see with clarity; things are exposed to you, but you must choose to look. If day of the week, see *Alphabet* for additional meaning.

DEAF　Closing ears to truth. You hear but do not understand, or choose not to listen because it means self-responsibility for change and growth.

DEATH　The old is dying; make way for new beginnings. Life is a process of death and regeneration into higher awareness, the old dying off in order for one to continue to grow. As blossoms die and fall from a tree, the tree continues to grow and change. Each little death actually strengthens the tree, for these are essential to total life unfoldment.

DEBT　As you sow, you reap, whether it seems positive or negative karma. Something you owe or that is owed to you.

DECAY　Negative thinking; unhealthy parts of self. Talents and abilities wasting away through lack of use. Examine, clean up, awaken to own potential, change to positive.

DECK　Extension of self, as a deck on a house. Exposed part of self to others. If deck of cards, see *Cards*.

DEER　Gentle, innocent aspects of self, often victimized by failure to awaken strengths and inner protection. See *Animal*.

DEFEAT   Results from pushing in the wrong direction or in the wrong way, one not in your best interest. A door is closed only for you to explore a better one. There is no such thing as failure or defeat, only opportunities for learning and growth. Ask what the positive lesson is in every experience; learn it and move on.

DEFECATION   Cleansing, purification, releasing, necessary to insure balance, well-being. Letting go of unneeded thoughts, experiences, ideas.

DEFORMITY   Part of self you have neglected or not allowed to grow into complete expression; fear of development and growth.

DELAY   Self-imposed restriction. Or, timing not right to go ahead. Also, fear of making the wrong choices; trust your inner guidance and move forward.

DEMON   See *Devil.*

DENTIST   Cleaning up verbal expression. Fear of pain and being out of control.

DEPRESSION   Low energy. Inability to see cause and effect relationships, how you are setting yourself up. Meditate and get clarity.

DESERT   Stagnation, no growth. Time to get on with your life.

DESIGN   Symbol, blueprint or drawing which suggests a plan or direction in life. May mean begin to examine your life plan, the big design or overall picture. Take a step toward your goal.

DESK   Problem you are working on; study, exploration, self-discovery.

DESSERT   Treating oneself. Each person deserves treats in life.

DETECTIVE   Searching for answers and insight.

DEVIL   Lower, ignorant side of self that tempts you not to accept self-responsibility, to blame others, procrastinate, dwell in negative thoughts and actions.

DIAL   Ability to transcend energy levels, tune in to different frequencies or thoughts with control.

DIAMOND   The many facets of the pure soul or self. Each learning experience, especially every seven-year cycle, enables you to buff or polish another facet.

DIAPERS   Be gentle with yourself as you release old programs.

DIARRHEA   Uncontrollable, unnatural releasing of negative thinking or fears. Flushing out wastes you have been unwilling to release, but now have no choice.

DIARY   How you see your life through own conscious perception; secrets, desires. A dream journal is seeing your life through the soul's eyes or higher consciousness.

DICE   What you are considering is a gamble, so think through the consequences before taking action. Look at context of dream for feeling level.

DICTIONARY   Search for knowledge; understanding of mental processes.

DIET   Searching for balance in eating habits; need for establishing balance in spiritual, emotional, physical, mental nurturing. Harsh or rigid diets reflect self-punishment. Moderation is the key.

DIM   Not seeing with clarity; you are getting only a glimpse. Raise energy level for clearer perception.

DINNER   See *Food, Eat.*

DINOSAUR   Ancient part of self; can be used creatively or destructively.

DIPLOMA   Initiation, graduation, job well done.

DIRT   Grounding. Putting hands into the dirt or earth has a healing, centering effect on the body. If a dirt floor, work on your foundation; if dirt road, your way is bumpy but will get you there. A large dirt area with no vegetation means a lack of growth in your life. If something is dirty, clean up your act.

DISABLED   See *Handicap.*

DISASTER   A fast, sudden change is coming into your life. See specific disasters for nature of the change: Blizzard, Flood, Earthquake, and so on.

DISC (Compact)   Clear blending sound that circulates energy and creates harmony.

DISCIPLINE   Self in role as student of life; we are all disciples, all learning. Specific disciple represents guidance or higher teacher.

DISCOVERY   New opening in awareness.

DISEASE   Disharmony; suppression of emotions that must be released in order for healing to occur. Stress and tension in physical, mental, emotional and/or spiritual life.

DISH   Self-nurturing vehicle; conveyer of spiritual food. Broken dish means denying a part of self that nurtures and serves.

DITCH   A diversion; depending upon width and location, creative thinking is called for to get around it. If walking in a ditch, you are locked into old realities, grooves, habits, that are preventing self-growth. A last ditch effort means poor planning and low energy.

DIVORCE   Rending apart, a severing of part of ourselves no longer providing positive growth. Understanding and letting go, necessary for a new beginning.

DIZZY   Going in too many directions, scattered. Need for balancing, centering energy. Caught in a whirlwind of action with little accomplishment.

DOCK   Place of rest from emotional seas of life; safe place for evaluating past and setting future course of action. See *Harbor.*

DOCTOR   Your inner healer; higher healing self. Guidance.

DOG   Masculine part of self; if ferocious means aggressive tendencies must be redirected in positive channels, verbalized.

DOLL   Depending on doll: if cuddly means a need for love and nurturing; if Barbie or Ken type means you are playing a role and suppressing true self.

DOLPHIN   Powerful, playful emotional, beautiful part of self. If we could learn to play in the emotional waters of life we'd never fear relationships and loving.

DONKEY   See *Mule.*

DOOR   Opportunity for self-discovery; if opened, walk through it; if closed, examine fear or block that is limiting you from going forward.

DORMITORY   Many parts of self are going to school, growing and learning. Diversities are being examined and hopefully integrated. Also, too much going on in your life: people, experiences, scattered energies.

DOVE   Mystical symbol for freedom, peace, spiritual awakening. See *Bird*.

DOWN   Wrong direction in life. Important to take a look at what you are doing and change directions.

DRAGON   Kundalini power. Fire from dragon purifies negative thinking, dispels illusion. Slaying the dragon means confronting and eliminating fears, enabling yourself to awaken higher level of awareness.

DRAIN   To release emotions. Also, see how you may be giving away your power, or losing your energy. Depends upon the context of the dream.

DRAPES   Closing off or covering up a part of oneself. See *Curtains*.

DRAW   Map out your direction; plan, create.

DRAWER   Storage place for ideas, available but closed off. If drawer is disorganized, time to clean out the old and keep only what is helpful, useful for present growth.

DREAM   To dream you are having a dream indicates more awareness in the dream state. When you become aware that you are dreaming, you can take control and ask any question you want to gain insight into yourself. This is a great opportunity to gain self-knowledge without the conscious mind intruding.

DRILL   To break through for opening to new insights and direction.

DRIVE   To drive and be in the driver's seat is to be in control of your life. Note how you are driving, and your position in the vehicle. If you are not in the driver's seat, ask who or what is running your life.

DRIVEWAY   Extension of self, making access to outer reality easier. Entrance to your house, or self. If someone else's driveway, see *Road*.

DROWN Warning; you are going under emotionally, over-loaded. Get clarity and perspective, lighten up; seek help if necessary. Emotional state must be changed. Time to relax, play, and not take the world so seriously.

DRUGS In positive sense, used to balance or correct dishar-mony within the body. Also, an escape from dealing with life, numbing oneself to outer conditions; searching for answers without rather than within. Looking for enlightenment through unnatural resources.

DRUM Pulse or rhythm of life. Heartbeat, brain waves. Com-munication, messages.

DRUNK Not seeing things clearly, you are numbing yourself. See *Alcohol*

DUCK Flexibility in handling emotional situations; adapt-ability in living—able to fly, swim or walk. If swimming with head above water, means you are on top of your emotions.

DUNCE Not using your head; think about what you are doing in life. Giving away power.

DUSK Ending of a relationship, situation or experience.

DWARF Short-sighted ideas; limiting your potential; not ex-panding into new areas of growth. Not seeing things in proper perspective.

DYNAMITE Caution, danger. Carefully examine what you have been suppressing. Open up, verbalize, deal with fears and emotions now. Seek help if needed.

EAGLE Great power; spiritual self is soaring. Tremendous freedom to be used wisely; accepting responsibility and taking care of own needs.

EAR Listen, pay attention, hear what is happening. See *Deaf.*

EARRINGS Important time for listening within to inner voice.

EARTH Mother Earth, the female God energy, receptive, nur-turing, sustaining. The womb of life, giving form and sub-stance to spirit. Experience of self in time; the earth embraces past, present and future. Humanness; temporal sensual na-ture. School for learning and growth; temporary home. See *Planet.*

EARTHQUAKE   Depending on magnitude of earthquake, a sudden big or little change in daily life. See *Disaster*.

EAR WAX   Not listening. Ears plugged up, not wanting to hear the truth.

EAST   Spiritual source, awakening; rebirth, as the sun rises in the east. Look within for spiritual direction.

EASTER   Spiritual rebirth; cycle of life and death as continuous unfoldment and growth. See *Resurrection*. If bunnies and eggs, represents a celebration, playfulness and delight.

EAT   Nourishment is needed, whether mental, emotional, physical or spiritual. You may need the specific food in the dream, or what it represents. See *Food*.

ECHO   Boomerang effect; self meeting self. What you send out comes back to you. Karma. Also, emptiness.

EGG   Closed in; living in a limited reality. Seed of new life, ready to open. See *Womb*. Used humorously, you laid an egg; reevaluate and clean up your act.

ELASTIC   Flexibility; also, stretched out, spread too thin.

ELBOW   Support, flexibility; essential for giving and receiving of energy. See *Body*.

ELECTRICITY   The life force; rate of vibration or frequency. You are an electrical being. Fuel needed for growth, clarity. See *Energy*.

ELEPHANT   Powerful part of self which can be gentle, helpful or destructive. Destructive only when frightened, so if elephant is angry, examine fears. Also, keep the positive lessons for growth, forget the negative dross of experience; you do not have to remember everything, even though the elephant never forgets.

ELEVATOR   Depending upon movement up or down, indicates whether you are going in the right direction. Moving up means going the right way, getting a higher perspective; down means going in the wrong direction. Down may also mean you are exploring deep-rooted problems, trying to understand your feelings and motivations.

ELF   Impish, fun part of self needed for enjoyment and entertainment.

EMERALD   Beautiful, majestic, healing part of self; durability, strength.

EMERGENCY   Wake up! Pay attention! This is an important lesson. Call for help.

EMPTY   Lack of self love, no energy; failure to use one's resources. Focus on creative self for new growth.

END   Completion. Let go of the old. Prepare for new beginning.

ENEMA   Cleansing, purification; releasing suppressed emotions, negativity.

ENEMY   Unknown aspects of self, those feared because misunderstood. At war within the self; befriend all parts of self through love, so greatest weaknesses become greatest strengths. See *Fear*.

ENERGY   We live, move and have our being in sea of cosmic energy. We are always in a state of either expanding or contracting our energy fields through our thoughts, words and actions. Physical, mental and spiritual levels of self are varying energy vibrations. Energy is the substance of our bodies and the fuel our bodies need in order to grow. Energy is the key to healing, insight, perception, and spiritual awareness. Meditation recharges the energy field, maintains its strength and state of expansion.

ENGAGEMENT   Commitment to self or another. See *Agreement*.

ENGINE   Power source, life force. See *Energy*.

ENGINEER   Fitting together, building, erecting new parts of self. If on a train you're taking charge of your path in life.

ENVELOPE   Covering or container. Indicator of news or message. See *Letter*.

EPILEPSY   Emotional suppression. See *Explosion*.

EROTIC   Desire for stimulation; fantasy, daydreams. Intensification of energy in the second or sexual chakra, active libido. Be more aware of body's physical needs and requirements.

ERUPTION   See *Explosion*.

ESCALATOR   Mode of quick and easy traveling, indicative of whether you are going in the best direction, making the best choices. If riding up, you are going in the right direction. If down, you are going the wrong way.

ESCAPE   Running away from self; if stuck and cannot move, you can no longer avoid working on the situation or problem. Running away in slow motion means you will soon be required to confront your fear. Remember to face what you fear and it will go away.

EUNUCH   Confusion of sexual identity; suppression of sexual feelings. See *Castrate*.

EVIL   Ignorance, lack of awareness. See *Devil*.

EX-HUSBAND, EX-WIFE   A man is the strong, assertive part of self. A woman is the, intuitive, creative part of self. Whatever qualities, characteristics, and lessons that you associate with that person you may be learning about again. Pay attention.

EXECUTION   See *Death*.

EXERCISE   Integration of body, mind and spirit; need to develop and focus physical energies. Relaxation, concentration. Get out of the intellect and play.

EXILE   Closing self off from all people and situations. Very low energy.

EXIT   Opportunity to leave a given situation; a choice.

EXPERIMENT   There are alternatives in living; examine new concepts and ideas, open up new opportunities. Try something different. May also mean you are taking a chance.

EXPERT   Teacher; one who has undergone lessons, is trained well, and who offers assistance. A part of self you may call upon for answers to your problems.

EXPLOSION   Eruption of suppressed negative emotions; important to deal with your feelings in a constructive way. See the hurts and make changes. Verbalize, release emotions on daily basis to avoid build-up.

EXTRACTION   To remove yourself from a situation; if tooth extraction, taking out an unhealthy part in order to establish harmony.

EYE The way you see things now. One eye represents spiritual self, the eye of God, expanded consciousness, clear seeing. Truth, power, clairvoyance. Both eyes opened means seeing with clarity; eyes closed means not willing to look at situations and lessons in your life. See *Blind*.

FABRIC The pattern of your life; you are the weaver of your experiences, creating beauty or chaos. See *Weave*.

F

FACADE Hiding from self; mask or shell you present to the world. Identification with outer values instead of inner resources and strengths.

FACE An unknown face may represent an unknown part of self, whether masculine or feminine. Also, face up to a situation; do not hide. A fogged over or unclear face usually represents a teacher.

FACE LIFT Creating a new face; a new way of looking at things. A whole new way of looking at life. See *Plastic Surgery*.

FAIRY Nature spirit; sustaining, helpful entity or energy.

FAKE Identifying with ego self instead of spiritual self. Pretending to be something you are not; blaming others for self-created situations. Covering up real self through fear. See *Mask, Facade*.

FALL, FALLING May suggest loss of control in a situation, low energy. Need to center through meditation to get back on target. May also be a "bad landing" coming back into the body at night.

FAMILY Integration of roles or aspects of self. Usually everyone portrayed represents you, although it could show you the dynamics of the relationship with a particular family member.

FAMOUS A famous person appearing in your dream represents your guidance or teachers.

FAN Indicates circulation of air, which is a change coming into your life. If face is covered or concealed behind a hand fan, you are hiding, need more self-confidence.

FARM   Nurturing, cultivating aspects of self. Working on development of potential; sowing and reaping. Growth is symbolized by what is on the farm and activity going on.

FAST   If moving or traveling at a fast speed, your life is full and encompassing many things; there is much for you to learn. Also, slow down and balance your energies. If you are on a fast, means purification and cleansing; also, self-denial and lack of self-love if carried to an extreme; destructive to physical energy.

FAT   Hiding from one's true self; poor self-image. Suppression of emotions, feelings; filling up with negativity and anxiety. Also, rich and abundant, as in the fatted calf, a fat wallet, living on the fat of the land.

FATHER   Wiser, more mature masculine self; the wise old man within. Aspects attributed to God, the protector and provider; or qualities projected on own father or father figure.

FAUCET   Ability to turn emotions off and on at will. Leaky faucet means energy is being lost through emotional worries; take stock of the situation and repair it.

FAX   Ability to communicate ideas, needs, and desires at a moment's notice.

FEAR   Being very close to truth and frightened to look at it. The other side of fear is insight. Seeing unknown parts of self and fearful of acknowledging them; resistance. Anything feared must be faced in order for it to go away. Your greatest fear is change; ironically, to change is the only reason you are here.

FEAST   A big celebration. You have done something well.

FEATHER   Lightness, uplifting thoughts. A feather in your cap is a job well done, talent or attribute developed.

FECES   Your own garbage, waste, unneeded attitudes and beliefs. Clean it up and discard it.

FEELING   The quality of feeling within a dream is important. Note whether you feel frightened, tired, confused, powerful, happy, supported, and so on. The feeling or sense of the dream helps you understand what you are working on.

FEET   See *Foot*.

FEMALE   Creative-intuitive, receptive, emotional, nurturing side of self; relatedness, feelings, the unconscious. That which is open, can be penetrated or entered. See *Male, Yin-Yang*.

FENCE   An obstacle which must be overcome before you continue with your lessons. A large, solid fence means give a great deal of thought to resolving your problem. A small fence, or one you can see through, will take less creative effort to move around, over or under it.

FERRY   See *Boat*.

FERTILIZER   The need for more meditation or spiritual nourishment to enhance your growth; a fertilized area suggests you are ready for insight, prepared for a new period of learning and unfoldment.

FEVER   Disharmony in physical, mental and/or spiritual being. Heated emotions which are surfacing in unhealthy ways.

FIELD   Place of rest, and relaxation.

FIGHT   Suppressed second and third chakra energy being released in destructive manner. Learn to verbalize and not suppress emotions.

FILM   How you see the past, which could be helping or hindering; usually old memories and your interpretation of life. Could also be a projection of the future, so pay attention to what you are creating.

FIND   To discover something new within yourself. See *Discovery*.

FINGER   Pointing a direction for you to follow. Pinpointing a problem. A finger of guilt at someone else means it really belongs to you; accept self-responsibility.

FINISH   Completion. You have finished what you began and new goals may be set.

FIRE   Kundalini or life force within, housed in the spine; Holy Spirit. Purification and cleansing of all belief systems so that you may open to higher knowledge. See *Kundalini*.

FIRECRACKER   Misdirected energy.

FIREMAN   Guidance, higher self. Part of self able to work with cleansing and purification, eliminating negative beliefs and attitudes.

FIREPLACE   Place of warmth and nurturing.

FIREWORKS   Depending on dream can mean it's time for a celebration of a job well done or your energy is being scattered and misdirected.

FISH   Need for meditation, spiritual food. The bigger the fish, the more meditation is needed. Also, something may be fishy, or not quite right.

FISHING ROD   Tool for spiritual and emotional growth; fishing for answers. Searching for spiritual awareness. What you seek lies within. See *Fish.*

FIST   Aggression, anger.

FLAG   Celebration of new changes taking place.

FLAME   Light of God within heart of self; beacon light for inner seeing, spiritual awakening. The more you meditate, the brighter your light.

FLASHLIGHT   Shining the light into the unknown parts of self. Look closely.

FLAW   Imperfection or destructive program within self, as a flaw in a fabric. Mend your ways.

FLOAT   If in water you have the ability to stay on top of your emotions. If floating in air you are in tune with the spiritual self.

FLOOD   Overwhelmed emotionally. See *Disaster.*

FLOOR   Foundation, support; that upon which you base your life. If dirt floor you are not building a good foundation.

FLOWER   The unfolding of flowers is a sign of good growth, a direction of beauty and fulfillment. The completion of a goal; a time of great achievement. Appreciation. See also *Bouquet, Blossom,* individual flowers.

FLUTE   Spiritual elation; joy harmony, melodious feelings and thoughts.

FLY   Insect means letting little things bug you; little annoyances.

FLYING   To dream you are flying means you are out of the body, freed from physical limitations. If you can gain conscious control of the dream, you may direct your movement and traveling to different locations in time-space. The waking state is really the illusion. Ask any question you want and the answer will be given to you.

FOG   Inability to see clearly; raise your energy to understand the situation or direction.

FOOD   Nourishment of physical, mental, emotional or spiritual self. See what kind of food you are eating. See *Eat*. Also, food for thought, ideas.

FOOL   See *Idiot*.

FOOT   Grounding, balance. Nerve centers and reflex points are in the feet, vital to conducting energy, balancing and healing the body. If injured on left, you are not allowing yourself to receive. If on right, you are giving away too much energy without replenishing it. Washing the feet means healing. See context of dreams. Barefoot shows that you are grounded and in touch with the earth. See *Body*.

FOOTPRINTS   Looking back over the past to see the positive lessons you have learned. Footprints ahead are the pathway to your success.

FOREHEAD   The eye of truth. We can see as God and our Teachers do if we can stay detached and in the third eye.

FOREIGN   New part of self not yet familiar to you, coming into being. If in a foreign country and dressed as the people there, may represent a past life in which lessons you were learning then are coming up again in your present experiences.

FOREST   Tremendous protection, growth, strength; entering the unconscious. If lost in the forest, means you cannot see the forest for the trees; take charge of what is going on in your life.

FORK   A tool for nurturing oneself. A fork in the road means choices must be made as to which direction you will now go in your life.

FORMULA   Solution to a problem is at hand. Develop a plan to accomplish your goals. Also, need to organize, plan and gain clarity on your life direction.

FORTRESS   Constructively, a place for protection and healing; destructively, a place to hide and wall off from people. You have a choice of moving in or out.

FORTY   Mystical number meaning the time it takes to totally recharge the body; period of rest, relaxation, cleansing and purification.

FOUNDATION   Inner strength, support, groundedness. The foundation of a house supports, maintains it. One's inner foundation must be laid on the rock of wisdom, understanding, and love. See *House*.

FOUNTAIN   Life, spiritual beauty; uplifting, rejuvenating, healing powers.

FOX   Sly, manipulative, slippery. See *Animal*.

FRAGILE   Great beauty within still in the process of forming, not yet firm in consciousness; vulnerability.

FREEWAY   Easy going. See *Road*.

FREIGHT   Excess baggage or trips you do not need. A lot of freight means you are trying to carry too heavy a load.

FRIEND   A quality you see in a friend is a projected quality of your own self, one perhaps not easily recognized.

FRIGID   Fear of emotional dependency on another; out of touch with body, sexually blocked.

FRINGE   Knotted up inside; or something extra or decorative that gives beauty.

FROG   Leaping from situation to situation without learning and without resolution. Used humorously, you have to kiss a lot of frogs before finding your prince.

FROZEN   Emotional nature closed down, energies locked up; immobilization. See *Ice*.

FRUIT   Reaping what you have sown; a job well done. Productive outcomes resulting from facing and moving through problems. Fruit of your labors.

FUEL   Energy needed by the body. If you are out of gas you are running yourself down. Take time to stop, recharge. If in a gas station, note gas gauge. See *Energy* and *Electricity.*

FUNERAL   Death of the old. See *Death, Burial.*

FUNGUS   Unhealthy emotions, disease, disharmony.

FUR   Protection, cover; instinctual nature.

FURNACE   Power. Where the kundalini is stoked to bring the energy up through the body. Power.

FURNITURE   Beliefs, ideas and attitudes that surround you. Extension of self; how you define yourself. Self-expression.

FUSE   See *Fuel, Energy.*

GALAXY   View of expansive self; interdimensional experience to awaken you to heightened awareness of self as creative energy.

GAMBLER   Taking chances; stop and see if you are working against overwhelming odds. See *Dice.*

GAME   The game of life, or game you are playing at present. See how you have determined the rules and possibilities for success. See *Stage.* Playing games with someone, especially in a relationship.

GANG   Unruly aspects of self; fearful attitudes and beliefs.

GANGSTER   See *Criminal.*

GARAGE   Place for resting, safety. Your vehicle should be parked in a garage only temporarily, or you are not getting on with your life and learning your lessons.

GARBAGE   Discarded ideas, attitudes and beliefs you no longer need. Negativity, trashy thinking that needs to be eliminated. All the trips and programs to clean up, eliminate, in order to build a positive, constructive life.

GARDEN   Fruits of your own labor; results of your work in growing and learning. A garden needs tending, watering, nurturing; a lot of weeds indicates you are not on top of things in daily life, so spend more time getting organized, sorting out priorities. Healthy way to still the mind, rebuild and recharge.

GARMENT FACTORY   Place for creating new roles.

GAS   See *Fuel.*

GAS STATION   Time to refuel and recharge your energy.

GATE   New opportunity, possibility. If opening the gate you are ready to move ahead. If gate is locked you are not yet ready; manifest new tools within yourself in order to move toward new beginnings. Ask yourself: what is the key?

GAUGE   Indicates the balance of physical, mental and spiritual energy.

GAVEL   Justice. The evaluative part of self may be getting your attention; consider a particular problem you are facing; or, something is now decided and you can dismiss the case or concern.

GEAR   Putting a car in gear is getting ready to go for new projects. Low or high gear is an indication of energy level.

GEM   See *Jewel.*

GENERAL   See *Guidance.*

GENERATOR   Motivations which cause one to start on a plan; energy of higher self to mobilize the will; incentive and urge to grow.

GENITALS   Creative and reproductive energy; source of maya or illusion. Sexual feelings, fears, hopes, identity. Masculine or feminine nature. See *Penis, Vagina.*

GERM   Small fears that are harbored; when energy or resistance is down, they take hold. Also, the seed or germ of an idea; essence of direction or purpose.

GEYSER   Burst of emotional energy, feelings coming up and out in a rush.

GHETTO   See *Poverty.*

GHOST   Part of self you do not understand. If someone who has physically died appears as a ghost, may mean inability to communicate with you clearly; or, some of your feelings about this person are not yet solidified. All beings are spirits whether in or out of the body, but a ghost usually suggests a haziness or unclear perception. Used humorously, means not a ghost of a chance.

GIANT   If a large, frightening giant, fear or self-doubt has grown out of proportion. Making mountains out of molehills. If a giant building, tree, or vehicle, indicates tremendous potential within you. Meaning depends upon context of dream; whether giant is threatening or magnificent.

GIFT   Form of initiation; pat on the back for a job well done.

GIRAFFE   Reaching for growth.

GIRDLE   Restriction; suppression of energy in second and third chakra; looking without instead of within to resolve problems.

GIRL   Female child part of self; usually the younger the child the more sensitive. May mean relax and play more, get in touch with your child. Girlish attitudes. See *Female*.

GLACIER   Closed down, frozen emotions. See *Ice*.

GLASS   If shattered represents the breaking of illusions, hopes, consciousness, dreams. See *Mirror*. Chewing glass suggests difficulty in verbalization; fear of communication with self or another; cutting remarks. For drinking glass, see *Cup*.

GLASS (Eye)   Enabling us to see with more clarity. If broken, your perception is changing to see things in a new way. If lost, you have lost your ability to see clearly.

GLASSES   Take a second look at a situation; you have better vision and can see more clearly. If wearing someone else's glasses, not seeing with your own inner eye of clarity.

GLIDER   Free floating, supported. The winds of change are upon you; you can ride through them and steer, flow, but cannot change them. Easy and simple if you relax and go with the flow. See *Airplane*.

GLOBE   See *Circle, Earth*.

GLOVE   Protection, cover. Avoiding contact with others; blocking both sending and receiving physical and emotional energy.

GLUE   Hold things together until you get more clarity; stick to it. Glued to a task, dedicated; solid, strong. To come unglued is to scatter your energy, lose perspective.

GNAW   Something eating away at you, bothering you, taking energy. Examine level of stress, anxieties, fears; rid self of extra burdens and negative thinking.

GOAT   Able to digest almost anything, which may indicate lack of judgment. Getting to the root of the problem; clean up negativity that is blocking progress. Using someone or something as a scapegoat, not accepting self-responsibility.

GOD   Love, Light, Truth, Creative Power; Wisdom, Oneness, Infinity. Higher Self, Master Teacher within all things and all people. All-encompassing love, total acceptance, power to manifest all things, beings, universes.

GOLD   Christ light, love. Something divinely bestowed upon you; great treasures within.

GOLDEN FLEECE   Initiation; spiritual message, divine protection.

GOVERNMENT   Working together for the betterment of our entire being.

GRADE   Stage of learning and growth; how well you are doing with particular lessons you are going through. If a grade in school, see number of grade.

GRADUATION   Job well done; ready for next stage of growth for you have completed your former learning assignments.

GRAIN   Seeds you have sown, work you have done. Spiritual food in life. See *Harvest.*

GRANDFATHER, GRANDMOTHER   Wiser, more mature masculine or feminine parts of self.

GRAPES   Nurturing for the soul; harvest of sweetness. See *Fruit.*

GRASS   Growth, nurturing, grounding, protection.

GRASSHOPPER   Hopping from place to place. Looking for growth.

GRAVE   The limiting depths one digs for oneself. Inability to take action. Creative thought mobilizes energy and helps one dig out again. Self has to propel self back into aliveness; no one else can do it for us. See *Death, Coffin.*

GREASE If in a car there's a need to get your life running more smoothly. Grease in a pan means you need to clean up your act.

GREEN Growth, healing, expansiveness, creativity. See *Color*.

GREY Fear, insecurity; lifelessness. Neutrality.

GROCERY CART An aid to help you accumulate and carry easily all the necessities for nurturing yourself.

GROCERY STORE See *Store, Shop, Market*.

GROOM The strong assertive part of self getting ready to merge with our creative/intuitive feminine side. See *Wedding, Bride, Bridegroom*.

GROUP Uniting different aspects of self.

GUARD Divine protection. If prison guard, a part of yourself, beliefs or attitudes, is keeping you imprisoned.

GUEST Part of self not used on a regular basis, but can be called upon when needed.

GUIDANCE, GUIDE Higher self, or advanced beings or mystical teacher guiding you on the path of life.

GUILLOTINE Get out of your head; intellectualizing, rationalizing, analyzing. Headless person means same. Intuition helps resolve problem.

GUINEA PIG Learning through tackling a problem, experimenting and taking risks. Positive symbol meaning one learns either how or how not to do something.

GUITAR Ability to create harmony or disharmony. How are you playing? Is tuning needed?

GUM (Chewing) Used humorously, you are in a sticky situation; watch where you step or you will get stuck.

GUMS Verbalization. See *Teeth*.

GUN Sexual energy. If shot notice part of the body that has been injured; you are losing energy from that chakra. If being chased by someone with a gun, you are fearful of own sexuality. See *Penis*.

GURU See *Guidance*.

GUTS   If spilling your guts you are getting things up and out; feelings. Looking at the truth of a situation, or the need to do so.

GYMNASIUM   Self-discipline through mental, physical and spiritual balance. May indicate exercise and raising your energy level.

GYPSY   Wanderer; does not deal with life in the here and now, but walks away from problems rather than facing them. If fortune telling, reflects own psychic attunement; or giving power away to psychic level of awareness, not tapping the mystical or higher consciousness. Any prediction or direction may be reviewed, accepted or rejected; you are in control.

H   **HAIR**   Power flowing from the crown chakra or higher spiritual center; the longer the hair the more power. If body hair, means protection and warmth.

HALLOWEEN   Costumes represent inner fears or desires one has not recognized. What one pretends to be or wishes to be in life; roles.

HALLUCINATION   Fantasy; not seeing things as they really are for fear of needing to change.

HALLWAY   A narrow pathway necessary to walk through; you can't get off the track. Whether light or dark reflects whether you are seeing clearly the nature of what you are dealing with. Passageway to insight.

HALO   See *Aura.*

HAM   Do not take life so seriously; ham it up a little. Or, you are being a ham. See *Food.*

HAMMER   An idea or tool, used to build or break apart. See how you are using it.

HAMSTER   Depending on dream can mean chasing oneself around and around with no direct goal.

HAND   Feeling, expressive part of self. Left hand receives energy, love; right hand gives. If injured on left, you are not allowing yourself to receive; if on right you are giving away too much energy without replenishing. Hand extended to you means help is available: look within, reach to others and to God. See *Body.*

HANDCUFF   Limiting self-expression; not freeing self to move ahead.

HANDICAP   Depending upon kind of handicap, one is limiting own growth by not recognizing potential or honestly examining self. See *Deformity*.

HANDLE   Having control of a situation; going forward by getting a handle on life. If broken, go within and find inner strength and resources; get a handle on who you are, what you are about.

HANG   To hang yourself is destruction through guilt and fear; lack of verbalization, choking off energy in the throat chakra, holding too much stress and tension. Release negativity, forgive self and others, and get on with the show. If hanging up clothes, represents your hang-ups.

HARBOR   Safety in an emotional storm. After rest and repair one must move out if growth is to be continued.

HARDWARE   Tools for building your life; ability to build, repair, mend. The nuts and bolts of life; glue that holds things together. Tools for knowledge.

HARP   Harmony, music of the gods; spiritual awakening or nurturing of higher self.

HARVEST   Culmination of work you have done on yourself. As you sow, you reap. See *Garden*.

HAT   The role or roles you play, how you present self to others which is not the full expression of who you really are. See *Cap*.

HAWAII   Relaxation, beauty, quietude, healing. Slow down and relax. Smell the roses along the way.

HAWK   To see and perceive from great heights; powerful; to soar spiritually.

HAZARD   Use caution. Examine your direction carefully.

HEAD   You are intellectualizing too much. Used humorously, means get out of your head. See *Face, Body*.

HEALER   Higher self, Christ within, inner healer. Wisdom of the self that corrects and balances, purifies and cleanses.

HEART   God force, Christ within; love, emotions, feelings. If cutting out a heart, means need to open feelings, love; have a heart. If being stabbed, you are losing energy through empathizing with others, getting caught in their trips; being drained emotionally. Rather than staying in your own or another's pain, always ask: what is the positive lesson for growth? See how you set up the lesson or situation.

HEARTH   Home, comfort; longing for or needing security. Going in too many directions; need loving support and regrouping.

HEAT   Strong emotions, desires, passion; as, a heated argument, or being in heat. See *Hot, Cold.*

HEATER   Need warmth, love and nurturing. Bringing comfort and love to oneself. Can mean you have turned off the emotions. Thaw out, open the emotions, and love.

HEAVEN   Many things to many people: reunion, rest, happiness, enjoyment, bliss, peace, enlightenment, understanding, love.

HEAVY   Carrying too much on your shoulders; get priorities clear, simplify, remove what is weighing you down. Delegate, lighten up.

HEDGE   Growth; if lining your pathway or road, suggests spiritual protection and guidance. If blocking, you are being hedged in; too many things in your life, conflicting ideas, demands on time.

HEEL   Vulnerable spot, as in Achilles heel. Heel of a shoe means you are being a heel. See *Body.*

HEIGHT   New opportunity and challenges. See *Cliff.*

HELICOPTER   Spiritual growth. See *Airplane.*

HELL   Difficulties one is going through; images in hellish environment suggests nature of problems. Fears to be faced and moved beyond. You create your own heaven or hell in the now of living. See *Fire.*

HELM   If at the helm, you are in control of your emotional life and can guide your way through stormy situations. If not at the helm, you are going up and down in the emotional seas of life, drifting, not accepting self-responsibility.

HELMET   Closing down the crown chakra. Depending on how it is used, can mean overprotective or just overcautious. Unwilling to get out of your head.

HEMLOCK   Truth; standing up for what you believe in.

HEMORRHOIDS   Lack of verbal communication, not loving yourself, suppression. Martyr syndrome.

HEN   Being a mother hen, overbearing, manipulative, protective. See *Chicken*.

HERB   Healing, soothing, energy; allow rest and nurturing.

HERD   Many parts of self. If rampaging energy is scattered; if moving calmly, energy is centered. Also, following blindly, not making own decisions.

HERMIT   Low energy; withdrawn. Need to be alone, get energy up; get out of limiting programs.

HERO   Celebrity or national hero represents guidance or higher self; otherwise may mean you have done something extremely well.

HERPES   Poisons erupting from within; if in the blister stage means have not yet eliminated source of problem. Suppression. Also, hidden sexual or other fears. See *Blister*.

HEX   Anger, hurt, inability to cope with a painful situation in a positive manner. Vindictiveness; hurting self or another.

HIDE   Afraid to deal with situations, not being honest with self. See *Hermit*.

HIKE   Recharge energy for clarity; physical and mental rejuvenation.

HILL   Opportunity for spiritual growth.

HINGE   Life hinges on perception; access to information and knowledge. Hinge swings in or out; it is your choice to open or close the door of opportunity.

HIP   Used humorously, means you're shooting straight from the hip. Learn to speak and verbalize your own truth.

HIPPOPOTAMUS   Emotional and physical weight; power through heaviness; lighten up.

HIT   Lashing out and criticizing self or another. Need for acceptance, self-love and expression of needs and feelings.

HIVE   Organized, productive use of energy.

HOBBY   Creative therapy, self-play; recharging and re-centering.

HOE   Tool for new growth preparation; used for breaking up limits, weeding out the negative.

HOG   See *Pig.*

HOLE   Dark hole is unknown part of self you are now facing. A hole in something means repair is needed; or thought processes are lacking, as a hole in your argument. Pitfall of your own making. If standing in a hole, see *Grave.*

HOLY   Holy Spirit or God-self, revered inner being, spiritual awareness. Something set apart as sacred or holy means lack of awareness. All life is sacred; God is the medium in which all things live and move and have their being. Something you have invested with power; return the power to the teacher within.

HOME   See *House.*

HOMELESS   Temporary lack of self-identity.

HOMOSEXUAL   Masculine part of self; merger of masculine qualities within the self. If making love with particular individual, may be merger within self of attributes associated with other person. Attitudes toward own sexuality. See *Sexual Intercourse.*

HONEY   Sweetness in life; abundance. See *Gold.*

HONOR   See *Award.*

HOOD   Hiding, inability or unwillingness to be seen as you really are. Deceit, dishonesty; protection.

HOOK   Getting hooked into something that may or may not be beneficial. Fish hook represents need for spiritual food; hook for hanging things suggests organization.

HORIZON   New beginning; clarity, wider view; expanded sense of self.

HORN   Warning; be aware, alert. Musical instrument means pay attention, see what is going on.

HOROSCOPE   Relationship of self to expanded celestial influences; life purpose and plan. Blueprint of life chosen before incarnation. What you do with it—changing, accepting or moving beyond—is own free will. Helpful guide or map. See *Astrology.*

HORSE   Freedom, power; sexual energy. Riding horseback suggests oneness with nature, expanded sense of self.

HOSE   If channeling water, emotional cleansing, feeding, centering. Conscious direction of energy. See also *Snake.*

HOSPITAL   Healing center; emotional, mental, physical rejuvenation.

HOSTAGE   Rejected or imprisoned part of self.

HOT   May be as simple as too many bed covers on while sleeping. A hot spot in your life that calls for cool emotional handling; you are in hot water. See *Heat.*

HOTEL   Large potential for growth. If seedy, need to work on self and clean up your act. If run down, you are not using your potential. If magnificent, you are rich in spirit and using your many talents. See *House, Building.*

HOUSE   The self. Where you are in the house and what is going on provides insight into the many facets of your life. Walking into darkened or unknown rooms is exploring unknown parts of self. If rooms are cluttered, get organized and clean out old, useless habits and ideas. Furniture and people in house are aspects of yourself. Note especially colors and shapes. Different rooms are different aspects of self:

Upstairs or attic – spiritual awareness.

Ground floor – daily living situations.

Basement – sexual awareness and unconscious.

Kitchen – work area, cooking up plans and schemes, preparation for nurturing.

Bedrooms – rest, dreams, unconscious, sexual feelings.

Library – intellect and learning.

Living room – daily interaction with others.

Dining room – sustenance, nurturing, fellowship.

Bathrooms – cleansing, elimination of the old.

Porch or *patio* – extended part of self, enjoyment, relaxation.

Foundation – inner strength and groundedness.

HUG   Comforting. Loving and nurturing oneself. Healing.

HUMOR   Ability to laugh at self, not take self too seriously. Laughter heals.

HUNGER   Hidden desires; need for spiritual sustenance, meditation.

HUNT   Looking for parts of the self, the unknown within you. Hunting animals may mean attempt to rid the self of animal or lower urges.

HURDLE   Limitation or belief to get over or around before continuing. Creative thought is the key.

HURRICANE   Strong, sudden changes. One is caught in an emotional storm rather than staying in the eye of calmness. Meditate and center.

HURT   Emotional hurt represents a truth being exposed you are unable to accept at the time; shattered illusions. You are always responsible for self; no one else can hurt you. Physical hurt means limitation; if bleeding from hurt, a loss of energy. See *Pain*.

HUSBAND   Masculine part of self. Qualities you project on husband. Perception of relationship with husband. See *Male*.

HYPNOSIS   Often suggests being under the influence of limiting beliefs about the self. You are hypnotized into believing you are a limited being. Buying someone else's beliefs instead of your own. Also, relaxation, meditation, expanded awareness.

HYSTERECTOMY   Eliminating the mothering role and going into a new stage of growth.

I   **ICE**   Frozen emotions and feelings, insensitivity; blocked from giving and receiving. You are on hold, immobilized, not growing. On thin ice means taking a risk; situation or relationship is uncertain.

ICEBERG   If tip of the iceberg, just beginning self-exploration; do not think you know everything: the more you learn, the more see you do not know. Drifting with no feelings. See *Ice*.

ICE CREAM   A treat; You've done something well. See *Candy*.

IDIOT Repeating numbers over and over, not learning from lessons; lack of clarity; making life much more difficult than it needs to be. Giving power away.

IDOL Worshipping false values and ideas.

IGNITION Power switch; turn it on to go and grow.

IMMACULATE CONCEPTION To dream of being impregnated by light or the God force means opening of spiritual consciousness; new beginning in awareness and opportunity for spiritual development.

IMPOTENCE Fear, insecurity blocking recognition of self-worth. Sexual impotence may be suppression; fear of own power, vulnerability; or reflect actual physical condition which is causing low energy and imbalance. Do not take self so seriously and play more. See *Frigid*.

INCENSE Sweetness; awareness of inner self connected with outer reality.

INCEST Merger of parts of self: adult with child, male with female. Two persons of same sex means you are embracing the feminine or masculine within you. All persons in dream are you; incest does not have to do with sexual behavior. See *Sexual Intercourse*.

INCUBATE Timing for new ideas not yet right; about to come into being.

INDIAN Teacher, higher self or guidance. Depending upon context, if being chased by Indians or any people other than own race, represents part of self foreign to you; you are fearful of that which you do not understand.

INDIGESTION Inability to stomach ideas, beliefs, situations, something going on in your life. Relax and evaluate the overload. See also *Nausea*.

INFECTION See *Disease*.

INHERITANCE Being given an opportunity, or gift in order to change your life. See gift or item received.

INITIATION You have reached a plateau; graduation. Awakening to new level of awareness.

INJECTION   Shot of energy; quick pick me up; healing. If addictive or lethal, you are injecting the self with destructive and dangerous thoughts; interference with the etheric body, blowing holes in the aura, losing energy.

INJURED   Stop and slow down.

INK   Means of creative expression. See *Stain*.

INSANE   Disassociation with reality, inability to discriminate. Sick, out of balance. See *Crazy*.

INSECT   See *Bug*.

INSULATION   Protection, warmth, preservation of energy, as when insulating a house. Also, hiding.

INTERIOR DECORATOR   Making one's life into an experience of beauty; changing, redoing parts of self.

INTERVIEW   Finding out more about parts of self; learning to integrate separate aspects of consciousness.

INVASION   Lack of privacy, need more space to call your own. Allowing negative thoughts to invade your peace of mind.

INVENTION   New way of looking at things; new idea for problem solving.

IRON   If ironing clothes, you are ironing out pressing problems. Also, too many irons in the fire. Strong-willed.

IRRIGATE   Balanced, controlled emotions, enriching and enlivening life experiences.

ISLAND   Refuge for relaxation, creative self-expression; closing self off from people; desire to run away from situations; isolation.

ITCH   Suppression, need to verbalize more.

IVORY   Purity; strength, endurance.

J   **JACK**   As tool for removing a tire, insures better balance and a smoother trip. To jack up one's spirits; elevate. Also, a jack of all trades may mean scattered energy, or healthful diversification.

JADE   Healing, growth. See *Jewel*.

JAIL   Self-imposed barriers resulting from inaction; key to getting out is creative thinking: define your goal and move ahead. Take responsibility for your life.

JAM Traffic jam means being locked into confusion, wearing blinders, not seeing the set-up. If spreading jam you are just making the mess bigger. Acknowledgment of power, responsibility, self-discipline needed to get up and out.

JAR See *Bottle.*

JAW If locked or closed, need for verbalization; release suppressed emotions. Sternness, strength. If jaws are crushing you, suggests fear of words, giving away power to others; losing control, being taken in by negative words of others.

JEALOUS Insecurity. Stop and work on self love. See your own beauty and self worth.

JELLYFISH Watch your emotional step; need for meditation.

JESTER See *Clown.*

JESUS Master teacher, higher self. See *Christ.*

JEWEL Priceless ability which lies within that you have not yet recognized. Undeveloped talent. Priceless gifts lie within you; recognize your inner beauty and creative tools for joyous living. See also specific jewels, *Treasure.*

JEWELRY Different gifts and abilities; adornment, beauty. Individual self-expression, identity. A particular stone may suggest you need that specific energy or color for health and well being. See specific jewels.

JOB What must be done now; stepping stone to growing and learning. Task at hand for developing specific tools of understanding. How you are seeing your work or job—drudgery or challenge, hard or fulfilling; your perception of your present work or attitude in life. To thine own self be true; to know yourself is to be aligned with the most fulfilling work, or creative self-expression, possible.

JOG Exercise; physical/mental integration. Also, escape from looking at self and relationships, responsibilities, as in just jogging along and not taking serious action for changes.

JOINTS Need to work together. Flexibility. Left is receiving side, right is the giving side.

JOURNAL   Daily ledger of experiences as a letter from self to self. Noted situations and thoughts may be used as lessons for growth or disregarded, depending upon awareness.

JOURNEY   Exploration of self; discovering new aspects of self through experiences in living. The life process from birth to death.

JUDAS   Betraying yourself. This above all: to thine own self be true. See *Prostitute*.

JUDGE   Depending upon context, may be guidance, higher self, conscience. Often indicates harsh judgment of self; you are your own judge and jury and must learn to be tender, gentle and self loving, in addition to being just and fair. If critical side judges self too harshly, you will also judge others harshly. Judging others. Whether self or others, judge not. Change what needs to be changed and move ahead. Lingering in guilt and condemnation lowers energy and insight level. See *Jury*.

JUGGLER   Trying to do too many things at once, scattering energy; playing role of super parent, super businessman, super spouse, or whatever. Concentrate energies because you are doing nothing well.

JUMP   To take a leap into something new. Move ahead. Also, look before you leap.

JUNGLE   Enormous growth. So much happening it's hard to assimilate it all.

JUNK   Old things and ideas no longer necessary to you.

JURY   Evaluative, critical self; fairness, clarity are essential. May be too harsh, unjust; key is balance in acknowledging where making mistakes and where on target. See *Judge*.

K   **KANGAROO**   Enormous power, strength. Huge feet suggest grounding, mobility.

KARATE   Learning to focus and direct energy toward desired goal.

KARMA   As you sow, you reap. What you give and receive from others.

KEEL   Emotional foundation. See *Boat*.

KELP   Emotional entanglements that slow one down in life.

KENNEL   Aspects of masculine self; aggressiveness, suppressed emotions.

KEY   Inner awareness that opens door to all truth; wisdom, knowledge.

KHAKI   Camouflage, hiding. Inability to see something clearly. Creating illusions.

KIDNAP   Stealing from part of yourself. If child is kidnapped, you are trying to take away your childlike nature. Examine how you are sabotaging your wholeness.

KILL   To kill someone or to be killed represents destroying parts of the self, killing off beliefs, behaviors or energies represented by the victim. If you are killing a parent, you are getting rid of some of your outmoded parental behavior or the old way of relating to a parent. If killing a child, you are destroying the child part of yourself or perhaps certain childish behaviors. Note whether killing male or female, old or young, and so on. Whether the aspects of self are useless and no longer needed or valuable and being denied, depends upon the dream context. If you are being killed and bleeding, you are losing energy or the life force. Your own thoughts, actions or others in your life are taking your energy. See *Blood*.

KING   Omnipotence, power; God. Wealth of knowledge, awareness of own self-worth, recognition of inner power. Ruler of your own life; self-responsibility. How you use creative power, wisely or foolishly, is your responsibility.

KISS   Affection, warmth, communication; also, the kiss of betrayal. See *Cupid*.

KITCHEN   See *House*.

KITE   Freedom to soar, spiritual power awareness; childlike awareness.

KNEE   Your support system. Need to be more flexible.

KNEEL   See *Bow*.

KNIFE   Powerful tool which can be used creatively or destructively. Cuts away unnecessary parts of self, as in pruning a tree. If being cut with a knife, may suggest surgical removal of unhealthy part; or cutting away parts of self still needed for growth and development. If being chased or chasing someone with a knife, represents fear, aggression, or energy loss. If bleeding, see *Blood*; also, *Kill*.

KNITTING   Mending, repairing, creating. Stick to the knitting; do not get scattered.

KNOCK   Pay attention to what you are doing; opportunity knocks.

KNOT   Tension, stress, as tied up in knots; closed off. Strength, unity, holding together.

KORAN   Spiritual teachings. Message from higher self.

KRISHNA   See *Guidance*.

KUNDALINI   Life force, spiritual power, Holy Spirit, God energy; housed in the spine and awakens seven chakras to full potential. See *Snake*.

L   **LABEL**   Branding or pigeon-holing something; suggests seeing the world through the eyes of separateness rather than unity. Feel the deeper meaning and connection of people, things, ideas.

LABORATORY   Work area to put together life plans and ideas; reflects where you are in life and how well you are staying on top of things. You are the alchemist, creating, blending life experiences to understand, transcend them.

LADDER   Step by step process of climbing to higher awareness. Way to reach new heights. If climbing down, you are going the wrong way.

LAKE   If water is clear, placid, you are in control of emotions; if murky or choppy, get centered and clean up emotional life. Emotional resources and sensitivity; not as powerful but more calming than ocean. See *Pond, Puddle, Ocean, Water*.

LAMB   Warmth, love, innocence. If slaughtered, means sacrificing thoughts, hopefully negative ones, to higher self. Better to give gifts of joy to higher self than to dwell on the guilt and sacrifice level. See *Sacrifice, Animal, Sheep*.

LAME   Condition or thoughts that are preventing you from moving ahead at full speed. Imbalance; limiting thinking. See *Deformity.*

LAMP   Light within. See *Light.*

LAND   Grounding, nurturing, safety from emotional turmoil. Foundation, solid orientation, depending upon appearance.

LANDSLIDE   Everything is coming down on you; feeling caved in. Pull back; you are trying to carry too much weight and responsibility. You are risking emotional overload. Stop and nurture yourself. See *Avalanche.*

LASER   Powerful, focused, concentrated energy.

LATE   Missing opportunities; undisciplined, irresponsible. Time is of the essence; be ready.

LAUGHTER   Healing, uplifting energy. Do not take yourself seriously; relax and enjoy self and others.

LAUNCH   Setting out on new adventure, discovery of self; aiming for a goal.

LAUNDRY   Cleaning up aspects of self; clean up your act.

LAVA   Unknown aspects of self, erupting after suppressed from consciousness. Message from the unconscious.

LAW, LAWYER   Guidance, teacher, higher self. Help available if you ask. See *Attorney.*

LAWN   See *Grass.*

LAXATIVE   Cleansing of the body; let go and release guilts, fears and hurts, suppressed emotions.

LEAD   Weight, heaviness in life. Burdened with unnecessary cares.

LEADER   Purposeful self, inner wisdom. Part of self that is leading you; examine whether emotional, mental, physical or spiritual, or integration of all.

LEATHER   Toughness, strength; instinctual nature.

LEAVES   Attributes; leaves on tree represent lessons learned, accomplishments, rewards. Fruit of activities. Many leaves mean great growth and accomplishment. Leaves on ground are things completed, let go.

LECTURE   Whether giving or hearing a lecture, it is teaching something; listen and remember.

LEECH   Someone is draining your energy. Stop and see who or what you're giving your power to. See also *Parasite*.

LEFT   The intellectual or rational; the left hand is the receiving hand.

LEG   Foundation in life. Motivation, mobilization that enables you to meet various lessons. Support system or ability to stay grounded. Left leg indicates receiving; right indicates giving out energy. See *Body*.

LEMON   Poor quality. Also, cleansing, healing agent. See *Yellow*.

LENS   Perception. How you see self and others.

LEPROSY   Wasting away of one's talents and abilities.

LESBIAN   Feminine part of self; merger of feminine qualities within the self. If making love with known individual, may be merger within self of qualities associated with particular individual. Attitudes toward own sexuality. See *Sexual Intercourse*.

LETTER   News or information; teaching.

LEVITATE   Rising above the situation. A lighter perspective. Effortless awareness and perception when you lighten up.

LIBRARY   Inner resources, knowledge. Learning new things; study.

LICENSE   Giving self permission to be happy, successful, take control of your life. Know yourself; dare to be you. Driver's license is your identity.

LIE   Inability to honestly evaluate oneself. Not wanting to see. Fear of truth.

LIFEGUARD   Guidance, protective higher self; safety in emotional waters.

LIFE RAFT   Staying above water in an emotional sea, but just hanging in there. Look at how you are setting yourself up and make positive changes.

LIGHT   Wisdom of God; power, energy, ability to see and understand. Christ light within.

LIGHTNING Forceful, powerful energy; awakening of kundalini or life force.

LILY Easter lily represents life, death and rebirth; process of growth and regeneration; transition. See *Flower*.

LIMB On a tree means ability or talent you have developed; each branch has own attributes or leaves. Also, hanging on by a limb. See *Tree*.

LIMOUSINE Enormous potential.

LINK Connection, part of the whole. You are a link in the chain of life. See *Chain*.

LION Strength, power, femininity. Fear of aggression, anger in self or others. Taming the lion is meeting one's own fears through inner strength and love. See *Animal*.

LIQUID Flowing, adaptable; ability to take on many shapes, aspects. Emotional, yielding, unstable.

LITTER Disorganization, confusion of ideas, uncertainty. Cluttered thinking. Prioritize, get organized, meditate. See *Garbage*.

LOAD Carrying too much weight, assumed responsibilities; unnecessary burden. Everyone could lift a lot of the load he or she thinks is important to carry around.

LOBSTER Get a grip on yourself.

LOCK Locked up inside, closed off; relax and open. There are no locks on the doors of heaven.

LOCUST Negative thought forms eating away at inner harmony; limiting your growth through gossip, negativity. Change to positive orientation toward self and others.

LOG (Burning) Having the strength to purify and cleanse areas of self that are destructive and no longer necessary in your life.

LOST Unclear on meaning, purpose and direction in life; indecisive. Lack of clarity due to low energy. Meditate and ask for inner guidance.

LOTUS Spiritual unfoldment. See *Flower*.

LOVE God is love. It is the greatest power in the Universe.

The more you love the more depths you open within yourself.

LOVER   Integration of masculine or feminine qualities within self. Desire for love, warmth, nurturing, self-acceptance, appreciation.

LSD   Expansion of consciousness, usually with no control. Awakening, expanded awareness. It is safer and more productive to use meditation, relying on inner direction, energies. See also *Drugs*.

LUMBER   Building material for your life. Getting ready to create new experiences. Strength, flexibility.

LUNGS   Purification. See *Heart, Chakra*.

M   **MACHINE**   Extension and utilization of natural power. If you become a machine you have lost touch with sensitive feeling levels, mind, body, spirit interrelationship. The body is an interdimensional temple, not a robot.

MADONNA   The Divine Mother in her many forms; mother of all. When the Madonna appears in a dream, healing is taking place. Feminine principle that unites with the Father God or masculine principle to bring the universe into being. Yin, the female, uniting with yang, the male. The mother principle within our own beings. Mother Earth. Mary is the personalized feminine divinity in the Christian tradition.

MAFIA   Conflict or war going on inside. Are you allowing others to manipulate you or are you using your power against others?

MAGAZINE   Brief portion of your life; reflections on a chapter of living. See *Book*.

MAGGOT   See *Decay*.

MAGICIAN   Trying to fool oneself or another; living in a fantasy world, trapped in illusions, playing games. Or, may represent the Tarot magician, with ability to transmute energy, being equally at home and in control of inner and outer universes. If pulling a rabbit out of a hat, you will need an ingenious idea to get yourself out of a situation, but you can do it.

MAGNET   Uniting, pulling together, in relationship, business, or other situation. Intense energy of attraction.

MAID   Nurture yourself more, take care of yourself and your surroundings. If depending too much on others to satisfy your needs, get back to yourself and look after your own needs. Don't be dependent. Also, need for a general clean-up of personal attitudes and everyday operation.

MAIL   Messages. See *Letter*.

MAKE-UP   See *Cosmetics*.

MALE   Assertive, aggressive, strong side of self. Rationality, practicality, intellect, consciousness, will. That which penetrates, understands. See *Female, Yin-Yang*.

MANAGER   Teacher or higher self that's guiding you.

MANDALA   Tool for focusing energy to center and balance oneself. A symbol of love.

MANSION   Tremendous potential within the self. "In my Father's house are many mansions," many talents, abilities and levels of consciousness you have not even begun to explore. As you learn to know yourself, the infinite nature of being, your true gifts, you will begin to utilize creative potential. Most of us are living in log cabins. Would you believe ant hills?

MANURE   Putting the past to good use; fertile growth.

MAP   Blueprint for life, the path you chose to follow, guideline, direction, showing you where you are and where you need to go.

MARBLE   A thing of beauty, yet cold and unfeeling.

MARCHING   All parts of self working together in precision and unity.

MARIJUANA   Relax and look within; draw insight and direction from an expanded level of awareness. Also, a dependency on outer stimulants rather than inner attunement. See also *Drugs*.

MARINES   See *Military*.

MARKET   Shopping around for new ways of seeing and doing. Everything needed is there, select what you want. Bringing into awareness new aspects of self. See also *Shop, Store*.

MARRIAGE   A uniting or bringing together of ideas, people, parts or aspects of self. To dream of marriage often represents a blending of the intellectual and intuitive or masculine and feminine parts of self. To dream of marrying a former lover or friend suggests integrating the positive qualities of the person into one's own consciousness, rather than projecting them on to the other. See *Yin-Yang.*

MARSH   You are on questionable emotional ground.

MARTYR   Lack of self-love; caring for others and not tending to own needs. Taking on responsibility of others, or causes, in order to avoid working on your own numbers. Cop-out; ego booster; "I have to do it all" syndrome. Release and forgive self and others; accept self-responsibility.

MASK   Different roles you play, faces you wear; not being true to self, dishonesty, hiding. Dare to be you.

MASSAGE   Healing, balancing. Physical, mental, emotional integration.

MASTURBATION   Need for release of stress or tension in the body. Take care of second chakra needs.

MATCHES   Tools for cleansing and purifying body, mind and spirit. Can also mean little things that ignite our fury.

MAYOR   Higher guidance or teacher.

MAZE   Confusion and feeling lost; a maze is always of your own making, often as a cop-out to avoid making decisions and accepting responsibility. If you are running around in the maze of life, imagine it changing into a freeway and get on with your growth.

MEADOW   Place of rest, relaxation, and safety honoring your growth and accomplishments. A period of refreshment and enjoyment before ascending the next mountain, your next phase of learning.

MEAL   See *Food, Eat.*

MEASUREMENT   Setting standards; your own expectations. Examine expectations of self and others. Rule of thumb. How are you measuring yourself? Is it realistic?

MEAT   Getting to the root of a problem or you may need to eat meat to stay grounded depending on the dream.

MECHANIC   Work to be done on your daily physical operation in the world. The body or physical vehicle may need attention, rest or repair.

MEDICINE   Healing, rejuvenation; balancing of body, mind and spirit. Also, getting some of your own medicine, karma. Correct your thinking.

MEDITATION   Know thyself; way to the guru or teacher within. To know the self is to know all things, God, the interrelationship and oneness of all beings, all life. When you truly know the self you no longer are judgmental of self or others, greeting all in loving acceptance. Meditation is the freeway to enlightenment; it keeps your energy field continuously expanding, accelerating your growth. It is so simple.

MEETING   Consideration of ideas, goals. Bringing things together. Integrating parts of self. See *Crowd*.

MELT   Opening of emotional resources, feelings; awakening to new understanding. Also, losing sense of self through taking on the heat of other's emotions.

MENOPAUSE   Freedom from codependency or mothering. Stop mothering the people of your life.

MENSTRUATION   Time of rest, cleansing, rejuvenation; relax and nurture the creative side of self. If bleeding is evident, see *Blood*.

MERCURY   Spirit, consciousness; changeable, unpredictable. Messenger of the gods. See *Planet*.

MERMAID   Spiritual and emotional temptation.

MERRY-GO-ROUND   Wheel of karma; you are going round and round in the same old numbers and programs. Take a look at what you are doing. Get off and make a little progress.

MESSENGER   Messenger of God; guidance, higher self. Listen to message for insight.

METAL   Strength, durability; hard, cold, unfeeling.

MICROPHONE   Verbalize your needs and feelings loudly, clearly, to be heard and understood. Not speaking up for yourself.

MICROSCOPE   Close examination of self; scrutiny. Getting a look at beliefs and limitations that are usually difficult to see.

MILITARY   If officer, represents guidance. If a military base, or you are in the military, indicates severe restrictions imposed on self. Giving away power to others rather than accepting self responsibility, determining own direction. Also, need for self-discipline.

MILK   Sustenance, nurturing; fulfillment, love, caring for developing parts of self. Milk of human kindness. Also, need for protein, strength.

MINE   Unconscious; hidden treasures within self.

MINISTER   Teacher, guidance. May reflect a role you or someone is playing, caring for others instead of attending to own growth, and working on own numbers.

MINK   Material values, luxury, abundance; protection, warmth, animal instincts.

MIRAGE   A false belief about self or others. Ego, projected illusions.

MIRROR   Self meeting self; seeing the world through your own programs and attitudes. Could also mean you are being critical of others and need to look at yourself instead.

MISCARRIAGE   Deciding not to go ahead with a plan, idea or program; aborting or releasing it because it is not the best way. Also, destroying a new aspect of self coming into being. See *Abortion*.

MISER   Unaware of own self-worth; lack, limitation. Not using talents, abilities, creative power. Selfishness through ignorance. The universe is abundant; you have only to tap its resources.

MOAT   Emotional block, defense against others.

MODEL   If fashion model suggests something you are trying to be or present; if a model of a vehicle or building, suggests planning, new development.

MONASTERY   A spiritual retreat, need to go within, explore masculine self and regroup before venturing into new lessons and experiences. Depending upon context of dream, may mean hiding from growth or calling in the world. See *Convent*.

MONEY   If change or coins, means changes are coming into your life; if dollar bills, big changes. Note any numbers and look up meaning.

MONK   Wise teacher. Depending upon context, may be one who is not in touch with sexual and emotional self to the degree needed in daily living.

MONKEY   If swinging from limb to limb, stop and get yourself centered; if chattering or jumping up and down, still the mind through meditation; if monkey is imitating others, recognize and change some crazy numbers you are running you have picked up from others. Monkey see, monkey do. Determine direction from within.

MONSTER   Fears of your own making, allowed to grow out of proportion through undue worry and attention. Any negative idea dwelt upon grows into something monstrous; it is but an illusion within your own mind. Make an effort to confront any monster in your dream; ask it what part of yourself it represents, what thought, belief, or fear. See the monster as a friend who has come to teach you something, bring you a gift. Picture the monster immediately upon awakening; imagine it unzipping its monster suit, and a little being steps out with a gift for you—insight. Remember all aspects of the dream are you.

MOON   Depending upon dream, security, inner peace, romance, love, quietude; creativity, inspiration. Also, emotional influence, as the moon affects the tides. If you are not centered, a full moon may increase feelings of confusion.

MOOSE   Powerful part of self.

MORTGAGE   A debt owed another; how you use energy to invest in experiences, borrow insight and time. See *Bank*.

MORTUARY   Represents those aspects of self which have died off or are no longer needed for growth. If you are sitting in a mortuary, means not growing or using your gifts.

MOSQUE   See *Church*.

MOTEL   Great potential to manifest your goals.

MOTHER   Usually represents older, wiser more experienced part of female self. Feelings you project on mother figure. If negative feelings, often reflects hatred or resentment of own motherly self which gives away power to others, lacks self-love, takes care of others needs and neglects own. See *Female*.

MOTORCYCLE   Need balance in your life; examine daily activities, schedule.

MOUNTAIN   Perspective, clarity, spiritual awareness. Seeing a mountain in the distance means enlightening experiences, opportunities, new lessons await you. Climbing up, you are going the right direction; climbing down means going the wrong way in some aspect of daily living.

MOURNING   Inability to release people, experiences or beliefs in order to make way for the new. Transition; open to receive new direction.

MOUSE   Little fear or irritant that is taking your energy. If cat is chasing a mouse, implies cat and mouse game with self or others; unwillingness to work on problems and resolve them. Many frustrating relationships are based on cat and mouse game plan. Quiet, shy, colorless, as a mousy person.

MOUTH   Verbalization, communication; express yourself. Also, a big mouth, a gossip; monitor what you say about others. Source for nurturing and sustenance.

MOVIE   This is your life; scenes depict current thinking, feeling, perception, relationships, and provide insight on problems. You are the producer and director; change what needs to be changed.

MOVING   Making big changes within. Growth and movement in becoming a whole being. Keep furniture (attitudes, ideas, beliefs) you like and discard that which is not necessary and outgrown.

MUCUS   Cleaning out suppressed energy.

MUD   If stuck in it, you are not moving or growing in life and need to get free of limiting thoughts and situations. If muddy or there is mud around you, clean up your life, your act.

MULE   Stubbornness; also, ability to carry a heavy load, but why would you want to play the martyr? See *Animal*.

MUMMY Wrapped up in your own programs, beliefs and habits; dead to the creative spirit within. Time to come to life through transcending your embalming fluid.

MUMPS Lack of verbalization; blockage in throat chakra, suppression. Storing up of frustrations, hurts, emotions. See *Disease*.

MURDER See *Kill*.

MUSCLE Strength, power, flexibility; strength by force.

MUSEUM Learning, knowledge. Integration of experiences. Also, out of the mainstream of life, outdated programs and beliefs.

MUSIC Healing, creative flow of life; joyful, uplifting. Inner harmony, peace, beauty.

MUSTACHE Power to clearly communicate.

MUTE Depending on dream it can indicate not verbalizing your needs or telling yourself to be still and listen more within.

MYSTIC God within, higher self, master teacher within us all. Through the mystical self you have the power to heal, counsel, teach self and others.

NAIL Protection for tender parts of self. Growth taking place. Depending upon how used, may represent a holding together, building strength and support; or, if chewing nails you are making life much harder than it needs to be, not seeing clearly; also hitting the nail on the head means the right perception, headed in the right direction.

N

NAKED See *Nude*.

NAME If you hear or see your own name, it means pay attention. If another person's name, represents qualities you associate with that person and need to actualize within yourself. Look up name under Alphabet and Numbers for numerological meaning.

NARROW Limited, restricted path; reduced options. May be a shorter route to achieve your goal, and discipline is required.

NATURE Haven for rest, rejuvenation and restoration of body, mind and spirit.

NAUSEA   Clearing and releasing the negative that has been suppressed; you have taken in too many experiences without understanding them, holding on to so much that you are making yourself sick. Get everything up and out, learn the lessons and move on. See also *indigestion*.

NAVEL   Connection to inner being; symbolic of spiritual or silver cord that connects soul to body. See *Solar Plexus*.

NAVY   Need for emotional self-discipline. See *Military*.

NEAT   Getting organized, cleaning up your act. Disciplined mind.

NECK   Sticking your neck out, taking a risk. Throat or fifth chakra. See *Throat*.

NECKLACE   Adornment of beauty and creativity within. See *Jewelry*.

NEEDLE   Creating, pulling things together, as in sewing. Something difficult to find, as the needle in the haystack. See also *Injection*.

NEST   Desire for family life, relationships, home base; safe place within the self. Need for own space. Incubation period, resting place, before new creative ideas emerge.

NET   As a hindrance, you are caught in the net or web of your own thinking and cannot see the way out; as a help, a net catches things you want, or can provide a safety when you are working on balance in your life (walking a tightrope).

NEWSPAPER   Message about your daily life, what is going on. Look at it; pay attention.

NIGHT   Not seeing things clearly; cut off from inner light of guidance. Moving into unknown parts of self.

NIGHTMARE   Any nightmare is a teaching dream, your guidance trying to get your attention. Nothing is scary when the symbols are worked out; it is just a way to get you to remember them. To dream you are having a nightmare is a double message to pay attention and get some insight. See *Monster*.

911   Wake up and ask for help! Important lesson before you. See *Emergency* and *Numbers*.

NIRVANA   See *Heaven*.

NORTH   Darkness, uncertainty, ignorance. Point from which you seek spiritual guidance. Cold emotions, feelings. If north represents up, going the right direction.

NOSE   Humorously, lesson is as plain as the nose on your face, but you are not seeing it; also, you are being a snoop, keep your nose out of other people's business. Detection of direction, following scent of a trail.

NOTEBOOK   Record of needs and wants; notes to self. See *Book, Journal*.

NUDE   Totally open and exposed, not hiding who or what you are. Good symbology.

NUMB   Cutting off feeling through fear; ask what fear is causing your retreat.

NUMBERS   Each number has a spiritual meaning, a special vibration, a symbolic message to you. Add numbers together to get your symbol (example: a 28 is 2 + 8 = 10, 1 + 0 = 1). Individual numbers are:

1 – New beginnings, oneness with God, unity of life.

2 – Balance of masculine and feminine energies; or balance in some area of living is needed.

3 – Trinity, mind-body-spirit harmony; dream has a spiritual message.

4 – Balance of energies with a partner; growing in perfect balance.

5 – Change taking place now or very soon.

6 – Guidance, White Brotherhood (teachers of truth); six pointed star symbolizing perfect balance of man, three chakras above and three below heart center.

7 – Mystical number marking beginnings and endings, cyclic periods for growth and development: 7 chakras, 7 days to create world, 7 heavens; every 7 years is death and rebirth cycle.

8 – Cosmic consciousness, infinity.

9 – Completion, ending of the old; triple trinity.

10 – New beginning with experience, a higher frequency of understanding.

11 – Power to creatively express dynamic balance of self; higher expression of 2. Master number.

12 – Powerful unit of energy; as twelve disciples, 12 months, 12 signs of zodiac. Cycle for growth and development. Also, meaning of 3, the trinity.

22 – Spiritual expression of balance and integration with self and others; higher level of 4, master number.

33 – Spiritual teacher; double trinity; master number.

40 – Mystical energy; time needed to totally recharge, renew the body; change to higher perception.

0 – Wholeness, perfection, as the circle.

NUMEROLOGY See *Numbers*.

NUN Teacher; spiritual qualities within the self. Celibacy. If dressed in black implies being closed off from material world; also, walled off from people. Black cuts energy and closes down chakras.

NURSE Healing ability, need for care and nurturing; depending upon whether nurse is male or female, may suggest need to nurture own masculine or feminine qualities.

NURSERY A brand new part of yourself has been born and now needs love and nurturing.

NURSING (A baby) Nurturing a brand new part of self with love. See *Breast Feed*.

NUTS New seed, potential for growth; time for preparation and working to reap dividends.

OAK Tremendous strength within. See *Tree*.

OAR Helps put you in control of your boat or emotional life; without an oar you are unable to steer and drift about. A guiding helpmate.

OASIS Emotional nurturing; refuge.

OBELISK Spiritual power, growth. Tower of strength. See *Tower, Pyramid*.

OBESITY See *Fat*.

OBITUARY   Death of the old: beliefs, programs, attitudes.

OBSCENE   Unacceptable or rejected parts of yourself; desires or images you do not understand in their symbolic form. No images are obscene once you look at the message behind them.

OCEAN   Sea of life; enormous emotional energy to be respected and used wisely. Source of your life force. If lost at sea, you are overwhelmed by emotions. See *Lake, Pond, Water.*

OCTOPUS   If swimming suggests perfect balance and harmony in emotional life, cosmic sense of self-propulsion as octopus has eight legs; if grasping at different things means going in too many directions without control; if emerging from the depths of the sea and appearing scary, means fear of unknown emotional depths.

ODOR   Quality of an experience, idea: an inviting aroma or unpleasant smell. If something stinks it is a bad idea.

OFFICE   Daily work life, productivity.

OFFICER   See *Policeman.*

OIL   Lubricant, healthful influence. Energy. Anointed with oil is to receive a great blessing. Pouring oil on troubled waters is to smooth out disharmony and disagreement. Also, an oily or slippery person.

OIL SPILL, OIL SLICK   Emotions are clouded and polluted. Clean up your act. Smooth out your emotional relationships.

OLIVE   Love, peace. Nurturing element with many uses. See *Food.*

OLD   See *Ancient.*

OM   Sound used as mantra, symbolizing God, Brahman, integration of all vibrations in universe. Attunement to God-self.

ONION   Seasoning life's experiences. If teary from onion, suggests phoniness; tears are artificial. You have not learned lesson from an experience.

ONYX   Unknown power and beauty which lies within the soul. Part of mystical superconscious. Black represents the unknown jewel, mystical quality within the self. Spiritual gift. With clarity, this light will shine.

OPAL   Translucent quality suggests all truths shine through. All facets of self, talents are available to you. Multidimensional. Great beauty.

OPEN   The way is being shown, things are getting clearer; a way out.

OPERA   See *Choir.*

OPERATION   Healing, repair; see what area of body, what chakra is being worked on. If a great loss of blood appears, means you should relax and protect your energy while rebuilding physically, mentally and/or spiritually. See *Body.*

ORANGE (Color)   Balancing of peace and energy, yellow and red. A blending of peace and love.

ORANGE (Fruit)   Nurture self. May suggest you need specific nutrients in orange. See *Food.*

ORCHARD   See *Garden.*

ORCHESTRA   All parts of self working in harmony.

ORGASM   If you reach orgasm in a dream, may imply you are not having an active enough sex life, or the need to release sexual tensions. This is necessary for body to stay balanced and healthy, and so often happens during the dream state. It is important to recognize that we are all sexual beings.

ORGY   Many parts of the self merging together, but in confusion resulting in waste of energy. Sexual energy is going in too many directions; stop and center your energies to avoid depletion. Over indulgence.

ORIENT   Being in the orient or any foreign place shows the awakening of a part of self not yet familiar to you. The East is symbolic of spiritual awakening. See *East.*

ORNAMENT   Something which helps the self feel good, adornment; on a Christmas tree suggests a spiritual gift.

ORPHAN   See *Abandoned.*

OSTRICH   Avoiding growth by refusing to face life. Sooner or later one must face the self; there is no permanent way to cop out.

OTTER   Playful, joyful part of emotional self; learn to swim with ease and playfulness through the emotional seas of life rather than fearing and dreading your experiences.

OVAL   New beginning, wholeness, completion; egg, womb, circle. See how used.

OVARY   Storehouse for new beginnings. Place of seeds of growth.

OWL   Wisdom; ability to see with clarity in the dark or recognize unknown parts of self.

OYSTER   Closed off; hiding from beauty within the self (pearl). See *Clam.*

PACK   If carrying a pack, represents the load you think necessary to haul around with you. See *Baggage, Suitcase.*

P

PACKAGE   To send a package is to give away a part of yourself, to project it on someone else; to receive a package is getting in touch with an unknown part of self. See *Gift.*

PADDLE   See *Oar.*

PAGAN   Undisciplined part of self; misunderstanding and misuse of energy, as the ancient pagan rites worshipping false gods.

PAGE   A blank page means you are not doing anything with your life; reading from a page means getting a glimpse of your life record. See *Book.*

PAIN   Suppression, avoidance of problem; disharmony in physical, mental, emotional or spiritual self. Note location in body, corresponding chakra, to determine problem. See *Disease.*

PAINT   Changing attitudes, cleaning up, redoing. Painting a picture is a new way of creatively expressing yourself. Note color.

PAINTBRUSH   Tool for creative self expression.

PAJAMAS   Role you play in the bedroom; also, sleep, rejuvenation are needed. See *Bed.*

PALACE   Magical kingdom within the self; great grandeur and potential.

PANDORA'S BOX   Process of growth: releasing all the negative, all fears, so positive awareness of self may emerge.

PANIC   See *Fear*.

PANTS   Cover for the lower chakras. Could be hiding your sexuality.

PAPER   Means for self-expression, writing; if strewn about implies get organized.

PARACHUTE   Help is here, guidance is watching and protecting you through your present experiences. Also, time to bail out.

PARADE   Many aspects of self; some you fantasize and some you role play; all you create.

PARADISE   See *Heaven*.

PARALYZE   Temporarily unable to function well, see clearly, due to fear.

PARASITE   Something or someone that eats away at you and drains energy; can be own negative thinking and fear, or relationship with another person who is sapping energy. See also *Leech, Vampire*.

PARENTS   Normally, your experienced, older parts of self. If parents have crossed over, could be an actual visit or message from them. See *Male, Female, Father, Mother*.

PARK   Place of beauty, recreation, rejuvenation. May suggest need for relaxation and taking time to smell the flowers along the way. Notice if park is well-kept, overgrown; how you feel there, whether peaceful or fearful. Reflects your awareness and experience of an extended sense of well-being and self-appreciation.

PARKING LOT   May mean you are parked and need to get up and get moving. Or, you are going too fast; stop and part for awhile, slow down your pace. Re-evaluate, look things over. See *Car*.

PARROT   Gossip; one who repeats everything and talks incessantly. Are you monitoring your mouth?

PARTY   Initiation, graduation, celebration. You have reached a new plateau, learned well; you and others are joyous.

PASSENGER   If a passenger in a vehicle, you are going along for the ride. Choosing to follow others' ideas and directions instead of your own; not taking responsibility for determining own life path.

PASSPORT   Ticket to freedom; you are free to be and do with your life whatever you choose. Create what you want.

PATH   Our direction in life. See whether going up (right direction) or down (wrong direction). See *Road*.

PATIO   See *Deck, Porch*.

PATTERN   Restrictive belief system; ways we handle ourselves in typically dealing with situations. Something to be changed and moved beyond.

PAUPER   One who is poor in spirit; denying own God self, gifts, talents, and opportunities to serve others. Not seeing self-worth.

PAVE   To pave or resurface is to make life smoother for yourself; taking the time to prepare your way before venturing ahead.

PEACOCK   Sign of beauty and pride. All the colors of the rainbow.

PEARL   Beauty formed within the self; beautiful, precious, strong. See *Jewel*.

PEDESTAL   Honor, recognition. Also, giving power away to something or someone, putting them on a pedestal. Ego or martyr trip, putting self on a pedestal. We are all equal beings.

PEGASUS   Inspiration. See *Horse, Flying*.

PEN   As writing instrument, ability to express yourself and communicate. If in a pen, you have blocks to overcome but they are not difficult. A playpen conveys a need for structured play time; be sure to get it in your schedule.

PENDULUM   Balance your life, as you are swinging from one extreme to the other in emotion and thought. Get out of the action-reaction pattern through meditation; observe self and others without getting caught in all the games.

PENGUIN   A flightless aquatic bird, represents self weighted down by emotions. Black and white indicates working with balancing energies, yin-yang, female-male, negative-positive.

PENIS   Procreation, power, aggression. That which penetrates, impregnates with ideas. Masculinity; feelings about body, sexuality. If seen through second or sexual chakra awareness, penis is given more emphasis and power than warranted. See *Genitals, Vagina, Male, Female.*

PENTHOUSE   The creative or spiritual part of self. Tapping into your highest potential. Perspective.

PEOPLE   Many different aspects of self.

PEPPER   Stimulant; hot ideas; heated emotions.

PERFUME   Sweetness, luxury; indulgence. See *Odor.*

PERIL   See *Danger, Risk.*

PERSPIRE   Emotional release, nervousness, fear; cooling down a heated situation.

PET   Self-chosen responsibility; something which nurtures us. See specific animal.

PHONE   See *Telephone.*

PHOTOGRAPH   How you are seeing things at this time; a picture to awaken a past memory because the lesson you are going through now is one you did not learn in the past.

PHYSICIAN   See *Doctor.*

PIANO   Harmony, balance, creative expression. If out of key, get in tune with yourself, what is going on around you. Eight notes on the scale represent spiritual awareness, uplifting of spirits. See *Music.*

PICNIC   Nurture self through play and relaxation.

PICTURE   See *Photograph.*

PIE   See *Circle, Food.*

PIED PIPER   You are playing and following your own tune, leading others down the same path. Make sure you are going in the right direction, emphasizing self-responsibility. If following the pied piper, you are being mesmerized by a belief, some aspect of self, ego, or another person.

PIER   Emotional safety region. You may stay for awhile to rest and regroup, avoid the ups and downs of emotional turmoil.

Also, you may survey emotional scene (waters) and gain perspective. See *Harbor.*

PIG   You or someone else is not sharing, being hoggish, whether with time, energy, money, or whatever. Hogging the credit which belongs to another.

PIGEON   Messenger; a message is coming to you, perhaps later in dream or in waking reality. Flight and freedom. As a stool pigeon, you are gossiping: monitor your mouth.

PILGRIM   One who is exploring unknown parts of the self; student of life. Searching for spiritual truth; look within.

PILINGS   Support. See *Foundation.*

PILL   Used humorously, you are being a pill; shape up your act. Also, you have created a hard pill to swallow and are in the process of taking your own medicine, or karma. As a medicine, represents healing.

PILLAR   Strength, support, leadership; independence and ability to stand firm in your beliefs and inner truths.

PILLOW   Bridge between conscious and unconscious; need for resting, relaxing the intellect and tapping deeper sources within self. Slow down your pace in order to see clearly, get insight. Tenderness, softness. See *Bed.*

PILOT   Higher self, guidance, the Lord, guiding your journey through life. Are you the pilot or is someone else leading you? An airplane pilot is in charge or your spiritual vehicle; a sea pilot is running your emotional ship.

PIMPLE   See *Blister.*

PIN CUSHION   Someone is sticking it to you; you are receiving the brunt of pointed remarks, harmful thoughts and attitudes; allowing yourself to be used. Or, you are wishing someone else ill through sharp words, negative thinking, and will only harm yourself. Need for repair. See *Sew.*

PINE   Tree that is highest conductor of energy next to the redwood. See *Tree.*

PIONEER   Exploring the unknown; looking for new ways of thinking, feeling, and expressing self, or the need to do so. See *Pilgrim.*

PIPE   Conductor of energy; each being is like a pipe, energy flowing through. Ability to tap higher levels of power, connect conscious and unconscious aspects of self. If smoking a pipe, suggests relaxation, unwinding, as in pipe and slippers. See *Cigarette*.

PIRATE   A part of yourself, something or someone is robbing your energy. See *Burglar*.

PISTOL   See *Gun*.

PIT   If standing on edge of pit, should take another direction. To continue brings darkness rather than clarity. If already in the pit, which is of your own making, realize that you cannot hide. You take all problems and concerns with you wherever you go. It is time to look at situation, uplift your consciousness, and get going.

PLACENTA   Aftermath of a growth experience; that which has served a purpose but which is no longer needed. Get the essence of the learning situation and let all the rest go.

PLAGUE   See *Disease*.

PLANET   Idea, understanding of great importance; teacher, luminary. Each planet has intelligence or vibration and is interconnected with all other heavenly bodies. Special vibratory rate in relationship to self and others; cosmic influence, energy, expanded awareness. Harmony of cosmic movement; purpose, design. We leave the body at night during the sleep state to study on different planets, incorporating the lessons each has to teach us; they are more advanced schools.

Sun – Light, truth, spiritual center, God force, Christ light; power, energy, masculinity. All life depends upon its light; pivotal force in our lives.

Moon – Unconscious, emotions, responsiveness, psychic awareness; femininity, intuition, creativity; reflector of light and truth.

Mercury – Mind, thought, communication, intuition, changeability; messenger of the gods.

Venus – Love, beauty, harmony, gentleness, emotion, femininity.

Earth – Growth, learning, grounding, time-space awareness; centeredness, compassion, creativity.

Mars – Activity, adventure, assertion, sexual energy; aggressiveness, hostility, passion.

Jupiter – Expansion, wealth, abundance of spiritual knowledge and expression, benevolence, luck.

Saturn – Discipline, learning, slowness of time and production; refinement.

Uranus – Awakening, transcendence, sudden fluctuations, changes, impact; extremes, unusual abilities.

Neptune – Unconscious, mysticism, inner self, psychic awareness.

Pluto – Consciousness unfoldment, transformation, spiritual expansion.

PLANT   Growth; depending on number, size and quality, represents aspects of growth in your life.

PLASTIC   Artificial; flexible, adaptable, insensitive.

PLASTIC SURGERY   Reconstructing and rebuilding for your self esteem or looking for love and self esteem from outside sources.

PLAY   To watch a play is to watch your own life. Remember you are the writer, director and producer; if you do not like what you see, you are free to change the script or produce an entirely new drama. If you are playing, or at play, rebuild creative energies, relax, and forget about competition and struggle.

PLOW   If soil is being plowed, you are making preparation for new growth. A need to prepare, make ready, for new experiences.

PLUMBING   Inner system of cleansing and release. If backed up, you are suppressing emotions, avoiding cleaning up your act.

PLYWOOD   Flexibility, strength, warmth. See *Wood*.

POCKET   Place for hiding; concealing part of self, identity from others. Something you carry around you think you need; place for safekeeping.

POEM   Inspiration, creativity; message from guidance.

POISON   Negative thinking; fear and judgment are greatest poisons you have to overcome.

POLICE   Help is available; guidance.

POLITICIAN   May be guidance, depending upon dream; also, someone or part of self is trying to sell you one particular way of doing things, not taking into account the many variations and possibilities available.

POLL   See *Interview*.

POLLEN   Spreading something around, sharing; fertile with new ideas. Also, irritant.

POLLUTION   Need to clean up thoughts, words and actions.

POND   Emotional reflection of self; quiet, not particularly ruffled by the winds of change, but boundaries are smaller. See *Lake, Water*.

POOL   Mirror; if swimming pool, suggests rest, relaxation, healthful exercise. See *Pond*.

POPCORN   When popped or popping means expansion of ideas, positive growth; kernels mean potential has not yet come to fruition. May also indicate a need for salt in your diet.

POPE   Guidance, spiritual teacher. Living by someone else's rules; listen to your own inner teacher.

PORCH   Extension of self; note furnishings, neatness, feelings. If an open porch, you are out in the open with what you are doing; if closed, represents another room of your house. See *House*.

PORT   See *Harbor*.

PORTRAIT   Painting of self as one sees self; if do not recognize portrait, is an aspect of self not yet known on the conscious level.

POSSE   All the strong, assertive parts of self coming together to accomplish a goal.

POSTER   See *Advertisement*.

POSTMAN   News or messages are coming, usually welcome.

May mean dream to follow is particularly important and will have information directly from your guidance.

POT   Signifies what you're cooking up, or making, in your life now. Examine condition of pot. Source for nurturing, creating. See also *Marijuana*.

POT HOLDER   Protection; be aware in your work, handle with care.

POTTER   Molder of your life. Create what you wish.

POVERTY   Not using potential or seeing your own self-worth. Poor in body, mind and/or spirit. Meditate, get your energy up and use your abilities.

POWDER   If a mixture, could be dangerous (as gun powder), medicinal or nurturing, depending on substance. If face make-up, suggests a cover-up, inability to see the beauty within. Humorously, may mean leave or make a quick departure, as in take a powder.

PRAY   Refining own awareness, getting clear on goals, needs and wants. God knows what you want, but you have to know in order to manifest it. Need for more spiritual time in your life; communion with higher self.

PREGNANT   Something new is coming into being; about to give birth to new direction, idea, plan, or higher awareness. If you want to be physically pregnant, this may be a message from your inner being you have conceived.

PREMONITION   To dream of a particular event that has not yet occurred usually is symbolic of your own self-growth. For example, to dream of a parent dying usually indicates that the old way of relating to the parent is dying or changing. This is a common dream among adolescents as they grow to their own adulthood. A predictive dream has a special feeling about it, and one learns to recognize this quality or level of awareness through experience. If there is a question, interpret the dream both symbolically and literally, and ask for further clarification in another dream.

PRESCRIPTION   Solution to a problem; getting clarity.

PRESENT   See *Gift*.

PRESIDENT   Your own leadership ability; guidance.

PRESSURE   Tension, stress, overload. Relax, unwind. Examine daily activities.

PRIEST   Higher self, spiritual teacher, guidance. See *Monk*.

PRINCE   See *Male*.

PRINCESS   See *Female*.

PRINTING PRESS   Repeating stories, situations or numbers over and over without learning from them. Also, communication, teaching.

PRISON   We live in prisons of our own making. See *Jail, Prisoner* and *Criminal*

PRISONER   See *Criminal*..

PRIZE   To win a prize means you have done well in handling a situation or learning from a difficult lesson; appreciation from higher levels.

PROBATION   To be on probation reminds that you have taken long enough to learn a particular lesson or to solve a problem. A probationary period has a limit. If you do not change, you will pay karmic consequences; for as you sow, you reap. Examine what it is that you have been putting off, changing or dealing with, and get it handled.

PROP   Tool for self-understanding; something which helps us along the way; supports, sustains. Props are temporary, and eventually are released through awakening insight.

PROPHET   Mystic awareness, guidance, higher self, teacher-knower.

PROSTITUTE   Misusing energy to get something you want. You prostitute talents and gifts by not using your creative ability to the fullest, compromising ideals. Dare to be you!

PROVERB   Wise teaching, message.

PSYCHIC   All people are psychic, so tune into your own abilities; manifest, create what it is you want.

PSYCHOLOGIST   The wise, understanding part of self.

PUDDLE Emotional nuisance; something within self that bothers you, that you can walk around, but you would probably be happier if you cleaned it up.

PULSE Beat of our life; rhythm, harmony. Strength of life force.

PUPPET Allowing others to manipulate you; giving away power. If you are working the puppet, you are trying to control and manipulate others.

PUPPY A new masculine assertive part of self. Needs love and nurturing.

PURGATORY Purification, cleansing. Examining negative programs and thoughts that have been limiting your growth.

PURPLE Spiritual protection; higher consciousness.

PURSE Your identity; if you lose your purse you are not sure who you are; may be giving power away to others; or transitioning into new self-concept.

PUZZLE Not seeing the whole picture, only pieces of your life puzzle, Thinking of life as a puzzle; lacking clarity. Center energies, focus, concentrate on the problem and the answer will be there.

PYRAMID Mystical power, initiation. You have done something well, passed a big test.

PYTHON Any snake is symbolic of the kundalini power, or life force within. If a python is squeezing you, your spiritual trip is choking you; you are out of balance. Don't be so wrapped up in the idea of spirituality. Physical, mental, emotional and spiritual are part of the one great cosmic energy. You must achieve balance before you can leave the earth plane. See *Snake*.

QUARTZ See *Crystal*.

Q

QUEEN Depending upon context of dream, may be guidance, leadership ability, or powerful feminine characteristics emerging in consciousness.

QUEST Searching for self in all the wrong places; look within.

QUICKSAND You are stuck in your fear and are going under with it. Get on top of it, expand your perspective, create an inner refuge of safety and harmony through meditation.

QUILT   Cover, protection, hiding; creativity. Depending upon context, may also mean warmth, rest.

R **RABBI**   Teacher, higher self. See *Minister.*

RABBIT   Hopping from one thing to the next without planning; lack of awareness in creation of your world. Cuddling and warmth; completion of a task with the speed of a jack rabbit.

RACCOON   Unwilling to let others see your intentions; not being totally honest. Eyes are clear seeing, yet masked for others to view.

RACE   If in a race, you are competing against yourself. Unite all aspects of the self in order to "win." If racing along by yourself, take some time to relax, integrate and reflect along the way.

RADAR   Energy, insight, attunement, intuition.

RADIO   Communication from guidance; message from higher self.

RAFT   Out on the emotional waters, but things can be shaky. See *Boat.*

RAGS   Clean-up time. Wasted ideas, energy. If dressed in rags, see *Poverty.*

RAILROAD   See *Train.*

RAILROAD TRACKS   You're on the track and you can't get off. Follow the self growth path.

RAIN   A cleansing in preparation for emotional growth; a heavy storm means changes emotionally, maybe tough ones, but it is only temporary.

RAINBOW   Perfect balance and harmony, completion, health, wholeness. You have come through difficult lessons and done a good job. Your higher self or guidance is well pleased.

RAM   Force, power, masculine strength.

RANCH   See *Nature* and *House.*

RAPE   You are losing energy, allowing someone's negative influence to take your power and self-esteem. Has no sexual meaning; do not take it literally. Simply indicates you are getting ripped off.

RAT   Betrayal of self; gossiping, judging others. Letting things gnaw away at you. Identify the problem and work to correct it.

RAVEN   Fear of the unknown. Flight into unknown parts of self. See *Bird*.

RAZOR   Mental alertness, clarity. Fine line between truth and falsity. See *Knife*.

REALTOR   One that's searching for new parts of self.

REAP   See *Garden, Harvest*.

REBIRTH   Spiritual awakening; birth of new ideas, insights, awareness of self. See *Resurrection*.

RECORD   You are playing the same old tunes, old programs, and going round and round. Not making any progress; sounding like a broken record. Look at your numbers, meditate, and raise consciousness so you can listen to your inner music.

RED   Life force, fertility, energy, passion; also anger, uncontrolled emotions. Lowest vibration in visual color spectrum. May mean you need energy. See *Color*.

REDWOOD   Highest energy tree; power, strength, wisdom. Grounded in physical reality yet ever reaching toward the heavens or wisdom from the higher self. See *Tree*.

REEF   Barrier to growth; caution. Also, protection while swimming in emotional waters.

REFRIGERATOR   Putting your feelings on ice; emotional coldness. Lack of affection, warmth.

REINDEER   Symbolizes giving part of self. If Rudolph, means let your light shine and dare to be different. Lead the way. See *Deer*.

RELATIVE   Aspects of self are represented by qualities or characteristics you identify with particular individual; rarely actually represents the person, but is almost always you.

RENT   Payment, debt, karma; agreement of exchange.

REPAIR   Something in need of repair; an aspect of your life needs working on, putting back together, mending. There is work to do; it is fix-up time. Clarity comes with recognition of the situation, determining action to remedy it.

REPORTER   To observe and perceive life in a conscious manner.

REPTILE   Cold-blooded. See *Snake.*

RESCUE   Depending upon context: if you are reaching out to be rescued, you are asking for energy and insight to resolve a problem. If you are in earnest, help is immediately forthcoming. If rescuing others, you may be sensing a need in someone else and seeking to be of service; or, you may be trying to save the world and ignore your own lessons.

RESERVOIR   Storage place for feelings, ideas, attitudes and emotions.

RESTAURANT   A lot of options for sustenance and nurturing; need for nurturing, communication, or fellowship of needs. If eating a particular food, you may need it, the vitamins and minerals or its particular vitamins and mineral content in your diet.

RESURRECTION   Understanding life, death and rebirth. Realizing that what we call life around us is but illusion; transcending the third dimension so that we may work on all vibratory levels. Enlightenment; ability to transcend dimensions at will. Awakening spiritual nature within, which represents the badly misinterpreted idea of the second coming. To dream of resurrection indicates resurrected insight, energy, awareness, selfhood, on many different levels, from any of various situations you have been going through.

RETREAT   Low energy, need for nurturing. When retreating from a situation, you do not have the energy to deal with it and need to recharge. Being in a spiritual retreat, or restful setting, suggests the need to go within and draw upon inner resources for renewal and understanding; healing.

REVERSE   Change directions; you are going the wrong way.

REVOLUTION   Something revolving, making a complete turn, means you are getting back on your path; you are at the

point of beginning with increased experience, more awareness. A partial revolution is a change in direction. A revolt
suggests you are having a war within yourself, usually between
the intellect and intuition. It is time for a change, and you
must be clear in your beliefs and what is guiding your life.

RHEUMATISM Closed down, lack of verbal communication,
suppression. Inflexibility in attitudes and unwillingness to
move. Examine your ideas and loosen up.

RICH Unlimited ideas, creative talents and abilities which lie
within. You have the skills, talents and abilities necessary to
create what you want in life.

RIDE If riding in a vehicle and someone else is driving, ask
who is running your life instead of self; or, what aspect of you
is guiding your direction. Also, you are being taken for a ride,
being deceived. See different vehicles. If riding an animal,
shows a oneness with nature, freedom, attunement.

RIFLE See *Gun.*

RIGHT The right side of anything indicates giving, creativity,
intuition, God awareness; going in right direction; you are
right.

RING Promise; eternal perspective. The ring of truth. See
Circle.

RISK Confronting a fear; opportunity for growth, to know
oneself. See *Danger.*

RIVER River of life; flow of your own life. If you are swimming against the current, relax and lighten up with the demands you have been placing on yourself. If you are trying to
get across the river and cannot find a way, you are temporarily
blocked in dealing with an emotional situation. Build within
yourself a new route, expanded perspective, in order to resolve
the situation.

ROAD Your direction in life. Examine whether paved, rocky,
or dirt; whether a two lane, freeway, or whatever; whether
winding or straight, going up hill or down. Conditions of road
suggest how you are creating your life at this moment. If the
road is going downhill you are going the wrong direction. If

going up and down, you are reacting to things in life, not making much progress, need to stabilize direction. If at a fork in the road, you are approaching a major decision. See *Crossroad.*

ROAR   Anger, aggression, fear; feelings emerging from the unconscious.

ROB   Losing energy. Stop and see who you're giving away your power to.

ROBE   A cover. Role in which we are covering up ourselves rather than opening up and daring to be us. Ceremonial robes mean that an initiation is being given to you.

ROBOT   Locked in intellect; unfeeling, mechanical responses to life.

ROCK   Strength, grounding, personal power.

ROCKET   Spiritual growth, unlimited potential; if taking off you are soaring into new heights of awareness; power. See *Airplane.*

ROCKING   Gentle way of raising energy to become centered in body, mind, and spirit.

ROLLER COASTER   Your life is going up and down. Stop and get balanced.

ROOF   Protection, depending upon condition of roof. Flat roof cuts you off from energy; examine structure and shape, such as dome-shaped, A-frame, and so on. Cover or necessary protection for crown chakra.

ROOM   Aspect of self. See *House.*

ROOSTER   See *Cock.*

ROOT   Support system, connection, into deeper levels of self; foundation. Deep roots mean standing firm midst the changes and elements of living. Feeler for support, nurturing. Root of the problem.

ROPE   Kundalini power, or life force. Strands of the rope represent intertwined physical, mental and spiritual being which is strengthened each time one meditates. Lifeline. If tied up by a rope, you are walling off the bound area. Free yourself by redirecting life energy into creative thinking and positive self-expression.

ROSARY   Form of meditation, focusing the mind to one point; need for centering, concentration.

ROSE   Love, beauty, innocence. The color rose signifies love. See *Flower*.

ROULETTE   Taking a chance; look at decisions you have made, what you are doing; you are gambling and may wind up where you do not want to be. Take responsibility for creating your best. Wheel of karma. See *Karma*.

RUBBER   Flexibility, insulation, protection; wearing rubber overshoes or rubberized garment suggests protection in an emotional storm.

RUBY   Precious love, great energy; fertility and expansion. Used in the middle ages by royalty for fertility.

RUDDER   Guide, steer; control of direction. See *Oar*.

RUG   See *Carpet*.

RUN   To run away from something means you are not yet ready or willing to deal with a situation; running away from aspects of self because of fear. If running in slow motion, you soon will have to face your fear, and cannot put it off much longer. To get insight: stop, face your pursuer, and ask for understanding. Facing a fear dissolves it, and removes a heavy burden of anxiety from your consciousness. If running toward something, you are eager to begin new growth and get on with your path. See *Race*.

RUST   Spit and polish time; there is work to be done within. Clean, shine up, those forgotten attributes and talents.

RUT   You are stuck in habits, beliefs, programs; boredom. Wake up and get out.

SABOTAGE   Self-destructive tendencies that block us from success and growth.

SACK   As container suggests concealment, hiding. Elimina-

S

tion of unwanted parts of self through conquering. If you are sacked in a dream, may indicate death of the old or giving away your power to others.

SACRED   Something sacred or hallowed indicates you have invested power into something other than your own inner teacher. All life is sacred. See *Holy*.

SACRIFICE   Martyrdom; you do not have to sacrifice your energy, ideals, and goals for self and others. All you need to sacrifice is the negative thinking and destructive tendencies (including martyrdom) that limit you.

SADDLE   Saddling yourself to an unnecessary situation. Also, protection and comfort, as when riding an animal.

SAFARI   Exploring unconscious or hidden aspects of self. If meet animals on the safari, see *Animal* or specific animals.

SAILBOAT   Emotional self; you are learning or need to learn how to navigate and flow with the winds of change, staying on course through the many currents in daily living. See *Boat*.

SAINT   Teacher, guidance, wise being, higher self. If particular saint, may be qualities within self you need to recognize at this time; or a special message from a higher teacher.

SALARY   The fruits of your labor; sowing and reaping. To experience the rewards of creative work gives us self-confidence, appreciation, strength. Contract. See *Money*.

SALESMAN   Open to changes, new ideas, ways of looking at things. Also, be very clear on what is right for you so as not to buy someone else's bill of goods.

SALIVA   Usually anxious to get started on a new beginning of some project or situation in ones life, hungry to get going.

SANCTUARY   Retreat within self for nurturing, healing and peace; very personal and necessary level of consciousness.

SAND   Limitless part of self, constantly changing, never the same, yet always there. Sands of time: all is illusion, nothing is permanent. Also, nurturing, grounding energy. If your house is standing on the sand, represents a highly questionable foundation. See *Beach*.

SANTA CLAUS   A humorous way of saying a gift is being presented to you.

SATAN   See *Devil*.

SATELLITE   Communication from higher self; moving into a new orbit. Spiritual awareness. Also, follower of someone else's beliefs; you are a satellite dependent upon another's energy rather than generating your own. See *Planet*.

SAVINGS   See *Bank, Money*.

SAW   Tool for building, pruning, to be used responsibly. Also, a tale, proverb, belief you have accepted or one that rings true for you now.

SCALES   Balance your life; see what direction scale is weighted, lightness or heaviness. If numbers appear, check meaning.

SCALP   Humorously used means to get out of your head; massaging it stimulates nerve centers for growth and relaxes us in the process.

SCAR   Emotional wound which has healed but is not yet completed or released. You need some work in releasing the person or situation.

SCARAB   See *Beetle*.

SCARECROW   False front, pretense, afraid of inner self and others. If symbolism from Wizard of Oz, implies you have little confidence in your intellectual ability; look within for own strengths and abilities.

SCARED   See *Fear*.

SCENT   See *Odor*.

SCEPTER   See *Wand*.

SCHEDULE   Restrictions placed on yourself that limit you; more important to go slowly and get it right. Unwillingness to make the right choices or to be attuned to the best cosmic timetable for personal growth. Completion of goals are important but not if it takes the place of learning your lessons.

SCHIZOPHRENIA   Primary cop out for self-growth; thinking it is easier to choose to walk around confused and in a daze than to take responsibility. Inability to function in or out of the body due to lack of balance, refusal to accept personal power. Lack of growth; no gains can be made because of unwillingness to function and inability to see with clarity. See *Insane.*

SCHOOL   Life is school; you are here only to learn and grow. You are taught by all people and all situations. Be enthusiastic; you are going to go through it anyway. Lessons never change until you learn them, so might as well get in and work through them now. Each night you are out of the body and learn in schools on higher levels. Each level of consciousness is teaching you something about the nature of self.

SCIENTIST   The rational, intellectual self; student of life. Also, guidance, higher self; wisdom, search for knowledge. See *Laboratory.*

SCISSORS   Cut out or get rid of what is no longer beneficial to growth. Fear of being cut by scissors means we are afraid of cutting ourselves off from part of the self. Cutting a picture or message out of a book or magazine means wanting to keep something that is meaningful to us, whether idea or ideal, and make it part of the reality of our lives.

SCORCH   Heated emotions; you are getting burned in a relationship, agreement. See *Hot, Heat.*

SCORPION   Stinging remarks, poisonous thoughts.

SCRIPT   Roles that we play in life. You are the actor, writer, producer, director of your life's story. You can change the script at any time. Anything not working, change the script.

SCROLL   Powerful truths. Your book of life.

SEA   See *Ocean.*

SEAL   Seal of approval; identity. Emotional energy, awkward but light-hearted.

SEAM   Binding together. Unity. Coming apart at the seams, scattered energy. See also *Sew, Needle.*

SEANCE   Sidetracking growth by getting stuck in the psychic level. Phenomena and contacting spirits does not help you live a better life.

SEASON   Each season has its own special significance in our growth. Each year the same lessons await us if we failed to learn them in the previous growing season. Also, represents the natural process of change, variation and progress in our lives; everything has its own season:

Spring – is the beginning of the growing season; we receive practical lessons in our relationships with self and others;

Summer – is a continued time of high energy and rapid learning;

Fall – brings a slowing of the energy and we harvest the insight from our lessons;

Winter – is a period of spiritual introspection, sorting, and preparation for the next spring of growth.

SEAWEED   See *Kelp*.

SECRET   Something you know but do not want to admit or share. Something hidden from awareness by your own choice. All secrets are within, but you have to be earnest in asking and really want to hear the answer.

SECRETARY   Helpful, efficient side of self. May reflect an overload of work or lack of organization; you need a secretary, the ability to identify priorities and accomplish what needs to be done.

SEDATIVE   You are uptight; relax, unwind. Take control, responsibility for self, rather than depending upon something external to self.

SEED   New beginning, potential. If you are casting or planting seeds you are building for future abundance. As you sow, you reap.

SEESAW   You are stuck in the same old programs and emotions, going up and down. Get off and get busy cleaning up your act.

SELF   Seeing yourself in a dream represents either past or present life roles. All people and symbols are aspects of self.

SELLING   Trying to motivate self to make a decision, take action. Could also mean you are selling yourself short, compromising yourself. See *Salesman*.

SEMEN   Creative ideas, power, energy. Masculinity. See *Sperm*.

SENSUAL   Feeling or experiencing sensuality reflects the need for TLC or nurturing the body; caring for the physical and honoring it. Getting in touch with own sexuality.

SEW   Repair, mending; creating something new. Binding together, integrating ideas and attitudes. See also *Seam, Needle, Pin Cushion*.

SEWERAGE   Old ideas and attitudes that need to be cleaned out. Belief systems no longer useful which must be let go. See also *Feces, Toilet, Urinate*.

SEXUAL INTERCOURSE   Merger of energies, aspects or qualities within self. When having sexual intercourse with a particular person, it represents blending the qualities of that person with self, and usually is not actually a sexual dream. Having intercourse with a member of the same sex means a merger of the masculine or feminine qualities within your own being. Could also mean you have a need for sexual release to harmonize and balance the body, this being accomplished through the dream.

SHADE   Protection, refreshment, as in the shade of a tree. If lamp or window shade, that which closes out light. See *Curtain*.

SHADOW   Fear, illusion, that follows you. Unknown part of self. Face the shadow and befriend it to understand the self-insight it offers.

SHAMAN   See *Guidance*.

SHAMPOO   See *Soap*.

SHARK   Powerful, imminent danger that threatens to take your emotional energy. Usually a caution: do not get in the emotional waters you are considering, or you will experience a substantial energy loss. Threat to your emotional balance. Take responsibility for self and act accordingly.

SHAVE   To groom, bolster self image. If shaved head, may represent acknowledgment of higher spiritual power. Also, a close shave or close call. See *Hair.*

SHAWL   Covering and protection for heart and or throat chakra. See *Heart, Throat.*

SHED   Storage bank. Ideas, attitudes and beliefs we have not yet decided to integrate into ourselves or let go. May represent a "holding pattern," that you are not going forward or backward. Examine what needs re-evaluating and cleaning out.

SHEEP   Non-thinking innocent trust, giving all responsibility for self to others. Develop the awareness of the shepherd or higher self within to protect and guide you. Also, lamb may represent desire for cuddling and sensitivity; a desire to return to innocence, which is an unrealistic and undesirable state. See *Lamb.*

SHEETS   Receptivity, openness, sensitivity, femininity; exploring sexuality, the unconscious. Clean sheets on the bed means a fresh start; you have cleaned up the negative. Sleeping on someone else's dirty sheets means taking on another's programs, vibrations, that you do not need. Note color. See *Bed.*

SHELF   An idea or to put something on hold that is not pertinent in your life right now.

SHELL   Holding feelings inside, pulling into your shell; closed off emotionally. Growth impossible due to non-activity. If an open shell, emotional nurturing. Cover, protection.

SHIELD   Protection. The white light shield of love can be used any time to deflect negativity, enable you to stay centered and balanced. Other shields, such as defense mechanisms, are only temporary measures.

SHIP   See *Boat.*

SHIRT   See *Clothes.*

SHOE   Grounding. Things which protect you on your journey through life. Do not judge another until you have walked in his or her shoes. Wearing too many shoes, filling too many roles. See *Foot.*

SHOOT, SHOT   To shoot someone or to be shot is harming or killing off aspects of the self. Losing energy or life force. To shoot a target is to aim for a goal. See *Kill, Hunt.*

SHOP   Variety of opportunities and tools necessary to grow are at your disposal. Searching for new roles to play in life. See also *Market, Store.*

SHORE   See *Beach.*

SHOULDER   Strength, power. Ability to assume responsibility, on your own shoulders. Aggression, to shoulder or jostle, push through. See *Body.*

SHOVEL   Clean up your mess. Shoveling dirt can mean planting new seeds for growth. If snow, breaking up frozen emotions.

SHOWER   Emotional cleansing; clean up your act. Let all the negativity wash down the drain.

SHRINK   Something is losing importance, power; deflated image of self. To eliminate the weight of fears, concerns, by shrinking them down to size.

SICK   Ridding oneself of toxins in the body; low energy. If throwing up, verbalize, get things up and out. See *Disease.*

SIDEWALK   Pathway. The smoother the way, the better trip you are making for yourself. An easier journey than on dirt, but not as fast as the road. See *Path.*

SIGN, SIGNBOARD   Signal, message. Pay attention.

SIGNATURE   Individuality, self expression. Look up name under *Alphabet* and *Numbers.*

SILK   Wealth and riches; energy conductor, calming to the senses, nerves. Sensuality; smoothness, softness, ability to flow.

SILVER   Spiritual protection; light, truth.

SING   Expression of joy, happiness, harmony; healing energy. Uplifts your spirits, raises kundalini or life energy. Praises to the Lord, or higher self, God, spirit of life.

SINK   If kitchen sink, clean up, wash up. You are too broad in considering a problem, are not getting the message, including everything but the kitchen sink. If sinking into something, you are going down into the muck and mire of own emotional state. Stop and make changes; you are headed the wrong direction. Release yourself of unnecessary burdens.

SIREN   See *Alarm.*

SISTER   Feminine part of self. Qualities in self you project on sister or sister figure. Perception of relationship with actual sister or person sister represents.

SIT   Look before you leap. Stop, relax and recharge your batteries before you go on.

SKATE   If on roller or ice skates, work on bringing balance into your life. You are sliding by responsibilities, not dealing with a situation, letting things slide.

SKELETON   Emptiness; spiritual deadness. Does not mean actual physical death, but that you are not in touch with feelings, emotions; unfulfillment. All that remains is illusion when we are out of touch with the spiritual self. Form without function. Body without spirit.

SKI   Play time; freedom. Also, bring balance into your life; you are going at a high speed.

SKIN   Covering, environment; facade you present to the world. Beauty is only skin deep; look within to spiritual values. Measure of emotions, feelings, as something makes your skin crawl, gives you goose bumps. Point of interchange between inner and outer realities; bridge.

SKY   The only way is up; lack of limitations. The sky's the limit. Move toward highest goal. Freedom, expansion.

SLAVE   Out of control, not taking charge of own life, giving power away to others. You may be a slave to beliefs, habits, ideals, other people's reactions. See *Addict.*

SLEEP   Lack of awareness. Unwillingness to see or change anything. Stagnation. Wake up! Also, if dreaming you are going to sleep in a bed, see *Bed.*

SLIDE   Sliding down is going in the wrong direction unless it's used as play. Rock or snow slide means things are caving in on you.

SLIPPERS   Roles we play. Pampering aspects of self.

SMELL   See *Odor.*

SMOG   Not seeing with clarity. See *Fog.*

SMOKE   Lack of clarity; things are hazy; confusion. Indicator of heated emotions; where there's smoke there's fire. Warning. See *Fog.*

SNAIL   Crawling at a snail's pace; not moving along very well with growth and learning. Break out of your shell and get on with it.

SNAKE   Kundalini power; life force, creative energy, Holy Spirit, healing power within. The kundalini is housed in the base of the spine, and moves up the spinal column awakening the chakras or energy centers. If snake bites you, means the energy is trying to break through in that particular area of your body. For example, if snake bites in the heart area, means the opening of love and feelings; in the throat, verbalization and communication. People often dream of snakes entering their bodies, which is the awakening of this energy; Snakes are a powerful symbol, never to be feared. Snakes represent the awakening or continuance of spiritual growth.

SNEEZE   Cleansing, releasing of suppressed emotions.

SNORKEL   Clarity and clear perception in viewing the emotional waters of life.

SNOW   Purity, truth, peace, relaxation. Untouched, virgin snow signifies new beginnings, a fresh start, a new look at your world. See *Ice.*

SOAP   Clean up your act. Cleansing of body, mind and or spirit. Take some time for cleansing, purification of attitudes, thoughts.

SOCKET   Plug for more energy. Meditation is your tool to recharge your batteries.

SOCKS   Warmth and comfort or roles that you're playing, depending upon the dream.

SOLAR PLEXUS   See *Stomach.*

SOLDIER   See *Military.*

SON   Masculine child part within self. Also, qualities you project on son; nature of relationship with son or person in that role.

SOUTH   Spiritual awareness; integrating higher awareness into everyday life. Also, slowness and relaxed way of living, as stereotypes of southern way of life.

SPEECH   If giving or listening to a speech, you are being given a message, teachings, that are helpful to your life. Verbalization, communication; express yourself.

SPEEDOMETER   Your speed of travel: too fast or too slow? Look at numbers on dial. See *Numbers*.

SPERM   Opportunities for new beginnings that may be accepted or rejected. If masturbating you are releasing energy, but not using it to create something new. See *Semen*.

SPHINX   Mystical awakening not yet expressed; must be awakened in self through understanding. Cold, hard, expressionless; lack of aliveness, turned to stone.

SPIDER   You create your own web or life space; you may go anywhere and weave any life you choose; the eight legs of the spider represents the cosmic energy for creating our own worlds. All too often we get caught in our own webs, forgetting they are but illusions of our own making; we seek to control, manipulate others, pulling them into our own limited realities. Trap; illusion; caution.

SPILL   Lack of awareness; scattered energy, not paying attention.

SPINE   Support; the most important part of the physical structure. Whether rigid or flexible determines your use of the life force, God force, or kundalini energy flowing through the body. The spine houses the kundalini, nerve centers, and is our key to well being and aliveness. If you appear spineless, or have no backbone, you are not taking self responsibility, standing up for your own beliefs. See *Body, Kundalini, Snake*.

SPIT   Releasing hostile, negative emotions; getting things up and out.

SPLINTER   An irritant, thorn in the flesh; negative attitude or habit that causes discomfort.

SPONGE   Soaking up everything, both positive and negative energies; not in control. Picking up everyone else's trips. Also, soaking up knowledge; very receptive, but need to discriminate, balance your intake. Sponging off other people's energy rather than generating your own.

SPOON   Tool for nourishment, but one spoonful is not much to sustain you. Born with a silver spoon in your mouth; high energy, protection, abundance.

SPORT   Your level of sportsmanship in life; how you play the game, operating above winning and losing, being a good sport or a poor one. Making sport out of love, playing at it, rather than working on your own numbers and growing within relationships. A particular sport may reflect need for exercise, self-discipline.

SPOT   Blemish, irritant, attitude that mars your thinking and behavior.

SPRING   Get some energy and bounce into your step; spring forward, grow, make a fresh start. Spring out of the old and into the new. Use your coiled up energy to undertake new projects. See *Season*.

SPY   Intruder; one who watches other people rather than getting on with own growth, putting more energy into how someone else is living instead of being in touch with own life. Fearful of how others will react to own ideas, plans. A watcher, not a doer.

SQUARE   Boxed in; too square, controlled. Balance in partnerships; see four in Numbers. Balance of our elements: earth, air, fire, water.

SQUIRREL   You have all the tools you need stored away; recognize and use them. Pack rat, squirreling things away. Doer; one who plans ahead.

STAB   See *Knife*.

STABLE   Protection for our power source. See *Horse*.

STADIUM   Huge capacity for all parts of yourself to join together in a team spirit for life.

STAFF   Support. Mystical symbol for guidance; steadying your way along the path of life. A shepherd's staff brings in lost or forgotten aspects of the self. Strength within own being.

STAGE   The stage of life. How you present or show yourself to others; beliefs, attitudes, behavior. Roles may change at any time. Your present performance. See *Actor*.

STAGNANT   No growth. See *Cesspool*.

STAIN   Blemish, disfiguration; something that needs to be cleaned up. If staining something, as furniture, note color. May be brightening up, redoing. See *Spot*.

STAIRS   Direction in life. Note condition of stairs, whether rickety or strong. If going up, the right direction; if down, wrong direction. Running up and down, you need clarity; make up your mind and get on with your life.

STAMMER   Unwillingness to verbalize feelings; hesitancy to communicate needs and wants. Insecurity, lack of confidence. See *Throat*.

STAMPS   To put your approval or reject some matter.

STAR   Light, direction, guidance, insight. Uplifting of spiritual insight, vision. Powerful energy; affords energy level, clarity to actualize goals, as when you wish upon a star. Symbol of own inner light that shines forth in the darkness; you are a light or energy being. The truth of your being.

STARVATION   Lack of love, cutting self off from life force. Nurture self with meditation, affirmations, relaxation.

STATE   Add up the letters and see *Alphabet* and *Numbers*.

STATION   A stop and possibly transition point on the journey of life. Here you may change destinations, or begin a new trip. Resting place for clarity, determining goals.

STATUE   Beautiful in form and dead in spirit. Frozen, lifeless.

STEAL   See *Burglar*.

STEAM   Cooking up new ideas.

STEEL   Strength, determination; inflexibility, emotional coldness.

STEEP   Indicator of great progress along path of life if going up; if going down you are headed the wrong way in a hurry.

STEER   To steer a vehicle is to take control of your life.

STEPS   See *Stairs*.

STEREO   Creating the greatest harmony and beauty that is possible.

STERILIZE   No growth. See *Antiseptic*.

STING   Little things are bothering you, as when an insect stings. Stinging remarks, thoughts. Clean up negative dribble.

STOCKINGS   Protection, support, warmth; helpful to foundation, legs and feet. As Christmas stocking, means openness to receive good gifts from the universe.

STOCKS, BONDS   Investments in self growth. Security lies within.

STOMACH   Emotional barometer, as when you cannot stomach something. The way you digest life's experiences. See *Body*.

STONE   See *Rock*.

STORE   Great inner resources; whatever the store, it offers variety and opportunity. New ideas, ways of looking at things. Inner wealth, talents, abilities. See also *Market, Shop*.

STORK   New directions; brings new growth, opportunities to you and drops it on you. Spiritual beginnings. White bird is a messenger of truth. See *Bird*.

STORM   Emotional downpour; many inner changes taking place; cleansing, purification. Suppressed emotions, fears, anxieties have surfaced. Release of frustration. Things look darkest before the storm. After the clearing, you will feel renewed.

STOVE   Warming up to new ideas. Cooking things up.

STRAIT JACKET   Restriction, limitation. Tied up in own conflicts; blocking creative energy and insight.

STRANGER   An aspect of self you are not yet familiar with.

STRANGLE   See *Choke*.

STRAW (Drinking)   Learning to direct emotions.

STREAM   See *Brook*.

STREET   See *Road*.

STRING   Stringing someone along, or someone is stringing you along. See *Rope.*

STRUGGLE   Making things much harder than you have to; there is no need to struggle and suffer. Flow with the river of life; relax and seek inner guidance. Inner confusion; struggle between parts of self.

STUDENT   Learning, studying along life's path. See *School.*

STUMP   Growth is cut off; plant a new tree. Some problem has you stumped. Try problem solving with your dreams!

SUBMARINE   Strong emotional support, protection; allows you to explore emotional waters and the unconscious with great protection and perspective.

SUBMERGE   Going under emotionally. Build your energy. See *Drown.*

SUBWAY   Discovering deeper aspects of self. If boarding a train, you're getting ready for a new direction. If changing trains, you're changing directions.

SUCK   Desire to return to the breast, to be cared for and nurtured without responsibility. Also, you are being a sucker, or sucked into something.

SUGAR   See *Candy.*

SUICIDE   Killing off aspects of self, creative spirit. Giving up, quitting, not tackling a problem. Self-destruction. Get your energy up and stop your negative programs. Warning.

SUITCASE   If packing, you are storing away problems instead of dealing with and eliminating them. See *Baggage.*

SUMMER   Play, growth, relaxation; freedom of movement, expansion. See *Season.*

SUMMIT   You made it; resolved a situation, accomplished a goal. Clarity, expanded perspective, intuition. See *Mountain.*

SUN   Christ, God within. Light of God, eye of truth. Power, energy, clarity, knowledge. That which brings forth life, nurtures and sustains. The light of your being. See *Planet.*

SUNDAY   Rest, attunement, spiritual rejuvenation. The number 1, as the first day of the week. See *Numbers.*

SUNGLASSES   Protecting my perception so I can see with better clarity.

SUNRISE   New beginnings. Energy is coming up.

SUNSET   An ending or closure of something in your life.

SURGERY   Cutting away unhealthy parts of self that are no longer necessary in order to heal. Note which energy center needs healing.

SWAMP   Feeling swamped with work; bogged down in emotional mire. No clarity or perspective. See *Marsh*.

SWAN   Beauty, grace, purity; ability to glide over emotional waters, yet soar to new heights. Perception, freedom, peacefulness of soul. On top of emotions. If black swan, the mystery of the unknown; appealing, yet not understood.

SWEETS   The sweetness of life; how sweet it is. Need for energy, quick pick me up. Treating oneself. Also, manipulative device: you cannot have dessert until you eat your vegetables.

SWIM   Learning emotional lessons; how to maintain and understand self in the emotional waters of life. Staying on top of emotions.

SWING   See *Pendulum*.

SWITCH   Power control; ability to turn on or off at will. Degree of control over energy and life experiences. If in a dark house and cannot find the light switch means your energy is down and you must get it up. New things are coming into being that are presently unknown to you.

SWORD   Truth, power; symbol of the two edged sword of karma: as you sow, you reap. Honor, protection, search for truth. Also, destruction, combat. See *Knife*.

SYRINGE   Cleansing device. See *Injection*.

SYRUP   Sentimental, excessive, or overdone emotions. You are putting it on awfully thick, to the point of insincerity.

T **TABERNACLE**   The inner temple of mankind, the Holy of Holies representing the soul or God self. See *Church*.

TABLE   Daily activities, whether working, eating or playing. To put off a decision, as to table a motion. Negotiation.

TAIL   Bringing up the rear, on the tail end; following, but not confidently or enthusiastically. Your past; experiences that are behind you. See *Back*.

TAILOR   Designing a new role for yourself; repairing or altering an old one. See *Clothes*.

TALK   See *Speech*.

TALMUD   Spiritual teachings. Message from higher self.

TAME   Acceptance of parts of self previously rejected; harmony, peacefulness within.

TANGLE   Lack of clarity on a problem, confusion; mixed up ideas, attitudes. Sort out the real issue; focus, meditate, get energy up for insight. See *Maze*.

TANK   A military tank indicates aggression, hostility, war; protection. A think tank is a storage or germination place for ideas. Stored energy, fuel, as in gas tank. Water tank reflects stored or suppressed emotions; heaviness.

TAPE   Playing your numbers over and over, stuck in the same old rut with the same old tune. See *Record*.

TAPE DECK   The subconscious mind, where all tapes are stored. You may play anything you choose.

TAPESTRY   Design of one's life; the many experiences woven together to create a life pattern. You see only the knots on the back of the tapestry until death; at that point you look at the design on the front and see its beauty and symmetry.

TAR   The unknown. Ideas from the unconscious expressed in physical reality. If tarred and feathered, means great hostility, aggression, self-condemnation.

TARGET   Goal, direction. Self-discipline required to reach destination.

TATTOO   Ego identity. See *Scar*.

TAX   Unnecessary burden you place upon self; self-judgment. Being stretched beyond your limit in a taxing situation. Taxing your energy and not rebuilding through meditation, nurturing.

TAXI   A temporary identity, you are in transition.

TEA   Stimulant, relaxation. Social interaction. Ritual of spiritual centering, sharing with others. Take time out.

TEACHER   One who shows the way. All beings are teachers, how to or not to do something. Pay attention to inner or higher teacher in order to make life simpler. You are awakened to insight by own receptivity; although all people are teachers, and a few are especially influential along your path, remember to be your own guru.

TEAM   All parts of yourself must work together in order to come out ahead in the game of life.

TEARS   Release of emotion, whether joy or sorrow. Emotional cleansing, release of sadness, frustration, suppressed negativity. Healthy form of balancing emotional energies. Spiritual awakening of love, oneness, inner truth; tears of awareness.

TEDDY BEAR   Cuddling, warmth, affection; need for self-love. Return to basic sense of loving unconditionally. Teddy bear does not hurt, rebuff affection, talk back. Also, immature aspect of relationship; you are in complete control with no give or take.

TEETH   Grinding up, tearing something into little pieces in order to digest it; beginning the understanding process. Strength, intention; put some teeth into your position. Discussion. Need to verbalize. If teeth are falling out, you are unable to understand a problem or situation; something is too tough to swallow.

TELEGRAPH   Signals you send and receive from others. You are always in the process of communication with the world around you; how well you stay centered and control emotions depends upon your energy level.

TELEPHONE   If you are making a call, you are asking for help or understanding in a certain situation; or it is necessary for you to do so in order to gain clarity. If someone is calling you, it usually represents your guidance trying to get your attention with an important message. Look at any telephone dreams closely.

TELEPHONE OPERATOR   Guidance. If you can't get through, you have to get your energy up.

TELEVISION Medium to get a better look at your own life, how you are dealing with situations. Communication with self. See *Stage, Movie.*

TEMPLE Inner temple. See *Church.*

TENNIS See *Game, Ball.*

TENT Temporary identity, attitude, belief, as a house is you. Impermanence, questionable foundation.

TERRORIST Uncontrolled sexual energy (second chakra); resentment, fear, anger, frustration due to suppression. Unguided, misdirected energy which will not resolve problem because it is within yourself. Look within through meditation and find the cause of your own pain. Redirect and control energy in positive, creative self-expression.

TEST Opportunity for growth and learning. Be aware of what you are going through; even seemingly negative situations are tests of awareness, whether you see the positive lesson and can move beyond them.

TESTICLE Power, masculinity; source of creativity. See *Genitals, Sperm, Castrate.*

THAW See *Melt.*

THEATER Life is a stage for self growth. See *Stage.*

THERAPIST One who helps us to detach so that we can see how we are setting up our own lessons. See *Psychologist.*

THERMOMETER Used as an emotional gauge, reflects whether emotions are cold, lukewarm or hot. If extremely high, you are in hot water or being hot headed. If used as an energy gauge, reflects motivational level and degree of clarity. If low, no insight or motivation. If high, perception and direction.

THERMOS Emotional container; keeps hot or cold feelings bottled up.

THIEF See *Burglar.*

THIN Flimsy, lacking strength and endurance. Also, agile, lithe, spiritually empowered.

THIRST Eagerness for knowledge.

THORN   See *Splinter*.

THREAD   Experiences woven into tapestry of life; ideas; a thread of truth. See *Sew* and *Weave*.

THROAT   Throat chakra is the source of verbalization and communication. If being strangled you are blocking verbalization, suppressing your feelings. Sore throat is need for balance in communication. See *Neck*.

THRONE   A seat of power.

THUNDER   Reminder of suppressed emotions, feelings. Warning of anger, hostility within. Aftermath of kundalini or powerful energy release.

TIARA   See *Crown*.

TICK   One little thing that's bugging you and draining your energy. See also *Parasite*.

TICKET   Opportunity for new experience; airline ticket, movie ticket, and so on. If a speeding ticket, you obviously are going too fast and need to take time out to relax, unwind.

TIDAL WAVE   Big, powerful emotional upheaval. Watch what is happening, resolve things, do not let them slide.

TIDES   Emotional fluctuations. See *Ocean*.

TIGER   Power, force; fear of own or another's anger. Femininity.

TIGHTROPE   Caution, awareness. Stay centered and balanced or you are in for a spill. People put themselves on emotional tightropes through fear, pressure, impossible schedules. You just as easily can walk on a highway.

TILE   Protective covering; cold, inflexible. Ceramic tiles may reflect creative expression.

TIME   Time is an energy which enables us to experience and refine our creative power. All life is dependent upon cycles of time; everything has its own season. From birth to death is the cycle of life, with many smaller cycles in between. We are continuously moving through the process of time; all is dynamic, changing; nothing is static. It is the perpetuator of illusion; all things dependent upon it are temporary, ever fleeting. To flow with life is to use the energy of time to its fullest; to effortlessly manifest our goals and desires. We are interdimensional beings, unlimited by time when we understand our higher nature.

TIRE TRACKS   Digging a rut for yourself. Usually means stuck in a rut.

TIRES   Mobilization. If have a flat tire, you are out of balance. Pump up your energy.

TISSUE   Cleaning up our own act. Need for letting go, releasing and cleaning up problems you're facing.

TOAD   See *Frog.*

TOE   Assistance in balance. Just beginning to get a toehold, a grip on what is going on in your life; grasp of the situation. Big toe may represent pituitary gland. See *Foot.*

TOILET   Elimination; cleansing self of unwanted and unneeded past experiences. Releasing, letting go, forgiving. If toilet is stopped up, you are blocking the cleansing process by hanging on to negative experiences.

TOMB   See *Grave.*

TONGUE   Ability to communicate, express yourself. If cut off, watch your words. Also, a sharp tongue does not turn away wrath.

TOOLS   Necessary implements to conquer all fears and reach all goals. All tools are within you for repairing, renewing, beginning again; learning, growing and manifesting what you want. Get to work.

TOOTHBRUSH   Clean out your mouth; gossip, negativity. Polish up communication. See *Teeth.*

TOOTHPICKS   Not verbalizing; things are getting stuck in your mouth, communicate with love and humor.

TORCH   See *Flame.*

TORNADO   See *Hurricane.*

TORTOISE   See *Turtle.*

TOTEM   Intuition; message from unconscious; spiritual identity.

TOWEL   Warmth and protection after a period of cleansing. Security.

TOWER   Spiritual power, point of clarity, vision. If locked in a tower, you are in the ivory tower of intellect, cut off from other aspects of self.

TOXIC CHEMICALS   See *Poison*.

TOY   Time to play, lighten up. When see your goals as toys, they are easier to manifest. The childhood spirit of play is your best creative tool; play with ideas and they happily take a new form in self-expression.

TRACKS   Path of growth to follow. Means you have to stay on this path and stick with it. See *Railroad Tracks*.

TRACTOR   Power to work on self; determine what you want to sow and reap, because you have tremendous power to get exactly what you ask for. Time to ready the soil for planting the seeds of insight. See *Bulldozer*.

TRAILER   If pulling a trailer you are lugging unnecessary weight. If riding in one, you are not in control of your life direction. See *Passenger*. If living in a mobile home, see *House*.

TRAIN   If in the engine, tremendous power to accomplish your goals. If a passenger train you are carrying many people, pulling them along, which may be an unnecessary weight. If freight train, you are moving with a heavy load. See *Passenger*.

TRAMP   Undeveloped potential, poor self-image. Wasted talents, abilities through lack of spiritual awareness.

TRANCE   If in a trance may mean spaced-out, not grounded or seeing things clearly. Also, tapping higher creative ability, insight, knowledge.

TRANSPARENT   Clear, easily understood. Transmits light, energy, so is easily perceived.

TRAP   Limiting, confining the self. Traps are of your own making; sabotaging yourself with doubt, insecurity and fear. Take back your power and dare to be you. Remember traps are illusions.

TRAPEZE   High minded ideas; daring inspiration. Swinging back and forth; indecision.

TRASH   Emotional garbage you carry around. Clean it up, straighten things out. Left over junk is best eliminated, not stored.

TRAVEL   Moving towards growth and self understanding.

TRAY   Need to nurture and serve self.

TREADMILL   Stuck in programs, attitudes, beliefs, going round and round with the same old numbers. Boredom through lack of growth. You are free to get off whenever you choose.

TREASURE   Wealth of talents, abilities, creative power within. Gifts of the spirit not yet realized. Inner gold, light or God force.

TREE   Symbol of individual growth, development through life. Roots are the foundation: strong and deep means connection with spiritual source; shallow is poor support, unaware of inner strength. Trunk represents the backbone, source of kundalini power, strength. Limbs are talents and abilities, opportunities for self-expression. The leaves are the many manifestations of your gifts, the results of flowering or producing in the world. The tree is responsible only for its own growth. Pruning brings more light and healthier growth. A scrawny tree means not recognizing potential, self-worth. Old gnarled tree means storms of life have taken their toll; one has not learned from lessons or pruned the unneeded parts. Be as the giant redwood, ever reaching upward in majestic self-expression.

TRESPASSING   Intruding on your own rights of self-expression; taking others' energy, or allowing your own to be imposed upon. See *Spy.*

TRIAL   Going through a test in your life. Need to remain detached to see what the lesson is.

TRIANGLE   Trinity; body, mind and spirit. Power, integration, balance.

TRICKS   Can be used humorously as a signal to lighten up; or running numbers on oneself.

TRINITY   Father, Son and Holy Ghost; body, mind and spirit; adult, parent, child aspects of self. See *Triangle.*

TRIP   Experience, lesson. If going on a trip, adventuring into a new aspect of self. Way one views situations; addictions and attitudes. A trip is but a learning tool, neither good nor bad. Eventually one learns to rise above all trips or investments in certain beliefs.

TRIPLETS   Three new beginnings coming into your life. See *Trinity.*

TROPHY   See *Award.*

TRUCK   Large, powerful vehicle. Great potential. If hauling, you are carrying an extra load. See *Car.*

TRUNK   Need to clean out and release old belief systems. See *Suitcase.*

TUMOR   Need to change a belief system that is not healthy for your growth. See also *Cancer.*

TUNNEL   Passageway through levels of consciousness to new insight, expanded reality. Tunnel vision is closed-mindedness.

TURKEY   Usually represents silly attitudes, unwise ways of doing things. Being taken into something, not using judgment. Feast, celebration, praise, as in Thanksgiving.

TURQUOISE   Healing, calming, peaceful; spirituality.

TURTLE   Slow moving, slow to make changes; pulls into shell with little provocation. Steadfastness. Shell is protection, safety.

TWINS   New beginnings, hopefully in balance.

TYPEWRITER   Means of communication and self expression. Need to organize and verbalize thoughts and feelings

U   **UFO**   See *Airplane.*

UMBILICAL CORD   Symbolic of silver cord that connects body and spirit. Nurturing; one is never severed or cut off from the life force, divine love and caring. Cosmic connection. Also, may mean dependency on person or belief system.

UMBRELLA   Cover, protection from emotional downpour. Sphere of operation. Belief system.

UNCLE   See *Male.*

UNDERGROUND   The unconscious.

UNDERWATER   Going into unknown emotional depths of yourself for understanding. A very healthy sign.

UNDERWEAR   Cover or protection of self. Part of self still hiding from true self.

UNDRESS   To expose your true feelings, ideas; not hiding from self or others. See *Nude.*

UNEMPLOYED   Not using talents or abilities through poor self-image or laziness. Lack of self-discipline. Out of touch with creative power. Low energy. Meditate, get energy up; get in touch with life purpose.

UNICORN   Mystical power aimed at the heavens.

UNIFORM   How you present self to others; rigidity in self-expression. Loosen up, gain flexibility and confidence.

UNIVERSITY   The opportunity to learn higher teachings. See *School.*

UNRAVEL   Discover, untangle; solving a problem.

UPHOLSTERY   Covering. To upholster is to fix up, renew, change one's image.

URINATE   Releasing emotional tension. Cleansing.

USHER Guidance is leading in lessons you need in order to grow.

VACATION   Time to take a break from cherished beliefs and opinions. go within and take a refreshing look at new and expansive inner resources. Time to play, relax, rebuild.

V

VACCINATION   Protection. Ability to go through experiences without concern or worry.

VACUUM   To vacuum is to clean up, remove dust and dirt. To create a vacuum within is to eliminate negativity, be ready for the new. Be sure to put in the positive. One cannot live in a vacuum, but must fill the self with creative thoughts.

VAGINA   Receptivity, openness; femininity, responsiveness. Pathway to safety for growth and development. Feelings about sexuality, body, womanhood. See *Penis, Genitals.*

VALLEY   Low point; peaks and valleys in our lives. Place of rest, relaxation. Opportunity for expansion, opening into new direction.

VALVE   Control point; regulator of energy or pressure.

VAMPIRE   Sucking energy from others, or someone taking your energy. Negative thought forms worry, anxiety, take away energy and power from the self. Each person is responsible for generating and maintaining own energy level.

VARNISH   Protection; beautification. Or, glossing over mistakes; superficial understanding. See dream context.

VASE   Means for growth. Display your inner beauty.

VAULT   Storing away valuables through fear; talents, abilities, locked up. Things you hide to keep them safe. The only safety is creative, abundant self expression.

VEGETABLE   Reaping what sown; balance, healthfulness in body. See *Food*.

VEGETARIAN   Self discipline through diet. Carefully choose sources of sustenance to maintain physical, mental and spiritual balance.

VEHICLE   You; your mode of self expression and operation. How large the vehicle determines degree to which you are actualizing potential. Whether you are driving or riding as a passenger reflects your degree of control and self responsibility. Color, shape and direction vehicle is moving up or down, forward or backward is important. See individual vehicles.

VENEREAL DISEASE   Disharmony and misunderstanding of sexual energy. Fear of sexuality. Misuse of sexual energy; imbalance.

VENOM   Poisonous attitudes; anger, hostility; lashing out due to insecurity, fear. Hatred of self directed toward others. Lack of self love.

VENUS   See *Planet*.

VETERINARIAN   Healing and uplifting our animal instincts, nature.

VICTIM   Unwillingness to take responsibility for creating own life. Martyr role. Inability to discriminate between what can and cannot be changed, to release the past and create anew. The victim role has to be left behind if you would truly find your life path.

VIDEO   See *Movie*.

VINE   Body or self. See *Tree*.

VINEYARD   Harvest of life experiences; fruits of your labor. The older the vines, the more they produce. See *Harvest, Garden*.

VIRGIN   Unknown parts of self; unexplored dimensions. Purity, wholeness. The myth of the virginal woman as the most desirable sexual partner is a limiting belief that harms relationships. It is in maturity, in the giving and receiving of love, that full expression of relatedness, openness develops.

VISE   Being squeezed to the breaking point. Check out pressurized situations in your life and loosen up. Force, holding.

VOLCANO   Eruption of suppressed emotions. See *Explosion*.

VOMIT   Spewing forth over indulgences; ridding self of excess, unnecessary ideas and attitudes you cannot digest or do not need. Getting things up and out. Need for verbalization; what you are holding in is making you sick.

VOTE   Your choices. You have a choice in every situation. Make good decisions.

VULTURE   Cleans up old parts of self, beliefs, attitudes, you no longer need. Feeds off old, decaying ideas rather than creative, new, alive ones.

WAGON   Vehicle without a power source, usually pulled by something. Load you are carrying around. If a toy wagon, may mean you need play to restore balance.

$\overline{W}$

WAIT   To everything its season. Time not yet right. Also, fear may be blocking insight, motivation to go ahead.

WAITER, WAITRESS   Male, female parts of self that nurture and serve. If mad at waiter or waitress, ask what part of self you are rejecting, not accepting. If service is slow, you are not allowing yourself the nurturing and sustenance you need.

WALK   Proceeding along your path; mobilization. See *Sidewalk*.

WALL   Block, obstacle. To wall off from others does not afford protection, only locks you in rigid roles and fear. Tear down a wall or go around it by changing beliefs, attitudes; risking, loving.

WALL PAPER   Sprucing up, redoing. Covering, hiding inner feelings, true self.

WALLET   Identity. See *Purse.*

WALRUS   Awkward self expressions, feelings, and emotions. Keep practicing!

WAND   Creative power within. You are limited only by restrictions imposed on the imagination. Inner reality can change instantly, thus changing outer reality and experiences.

WAR   Fighting within self; rejecting parts of self. All aspects must work in harmony; intellect, intuition, male-female, body, mind, spirit. Need for balance, integration.

WARDEN   Critical part of self. Disciplinarian. Controlling, restrictive; loss of self power.

WARDROBE   See *Clothes.*

WAREHOUSE   Storage bank of ideas and talents within the self, seldom used. Tremendous potential; everything you want or need is there.

WARM   Depending upon context, safe, comfortable, feeling, affection. Balance of emotional temperature, neither too hot nor too cold.

WARN   Caution; watch what you are getting involved with. Dream may explain situation to be aware of.

WART   Something no longer needed that can be cut away, removed. Hard, callused part of self not needed for growth.

WASH   Clean up your act; cleansing, purification of emotions.

WASP   See *Bee.*

WATCH   If watching or observing a situation, you are learning lessons vicariously. Integrate importance, essence in own life. See *Clock.*

WATER   Emotional energy. Whether clean, murky, still or choppy shows emotional state.

WATERFALL   Electromagnetic energy that feeds and heals. Releasing and expression of emotions in healthful way.

WAVE   To be riding a wave is moving on powerful feelings, emotions. Sitting on the shore watching waves suggests drawing energy into self for renewal and recharging. Changes, going up and down. To wave at someone is acknowledgment, greeting, love.

WAX   Soft, impressionable, easily molded. Cleans and polishes; creates a shiny surface.

WEAK   Giving away power to others. Refusal to recognize own potential and self worth.

WEALTH   Knowledge, wisdom, understanding, creative power. The wealth of ideas to achieve desired goals is within.

WEAPON   Misuse of energy; defense, control, manipulation. Words may be weapons. Insight and love are the only weapons needed to create the kind of world we want. See *Gun.*

WEATHER   Emotional temperament; flow of good or bad fortune in life. Of course, you are creating the flow.

WEAVE   Putting together the many experiences of life into a completeness, wholeness. Blending effort, insight and direction to create the life you want. See *Tapestry.*

WEB   Network or entanglement. See *Spider.*

WEDDING   See *Marriage.*

WEDDING VEIL   A beautiful merger and union is taking place within you. A very beautiful sign.

WEED   Bad habit to eliminate in your garden of life.

WEEK   Unit of time. See *Time, Numbers* (7).

WELL   Reservoir, source of inner feelings. Way to get trapped emotions up and out. A wishing well conveys idea that emotional desire, (concentrated) focusing on the wish and expectation will actualize hopes and dreams.

WEREWOLF   Aggression, anger, fear; lower or animal urges within self. See *Monster.*

WEST   Exploration, adventure, unconscious or unknown aspects of self.

WETSUIT   Protection when exploring emotional waters or unconscious parts of self.

WHALE   Emotional power. Perception, intuition. Whale of an opportunity is coming.

WHEAT   See *Grain.*

WHEEL   Wheel of life, eternal circle; self meeting self. Wheel of fortune. Wheel of karma; the merry-go-round of sowing and reaping. Also, ease in getting around; mobilization.

WHIP   Verbal whipping of self or others; self punishment. Aggression, hostility.

WHISKERS   Growth, protection. See *Beard.*

WHISPER   Lacking clarity in communication. Holding self back; fear of full expression. Passivity; hiding secrets, not open. Dare to be you.

WHISTLE   Attention.

WHITE   Truth, purity, light of God, Christ light, protection, guidance.

WHORE   See *Prostitute.*

WIDOW   Male attributes within self have died off through lack of development or use. Bring in more masculine strengths; achieve balance. See *Male.*

WIDOWER   Bring in more feminine aspects; achieve balance. See *Female.*

WIFE   Feminine part of self. See *Female.*

WIG   Different ways of using power.

WILL   Clarity, motivation, direction. If writing a will, time to take an overview of your life; make concrete decisions. Put together things that are of value within the self. The act of finalizing something makes one stop and carefully review it. Take a look at what your life is about, what you want to accomplish, give to self and others.

WIND   Change. Strong wind is big changes; light wind is small ones.

WINDOW   Ability to see beyond a given situation; expanded vision, perception. Window to the other side, interdimensional awareness. House without windows is a prison.

WINE   Celebration, relaxation. Essence of life's experiences, the wine of life. Spiritual attunement; wine represents the blood or spiritual life energy of the Christ within. Communion with self, others, God.

WINGS   Freedom. Soar to new heights. No limitations. Through awakening spiritual consciousness there is nothing you cannot achieve.

WINTER   See *Season*.

WIRE   Support. Pliable, dependable strength. Ability to repair, mend a situation. Humorously, may mean you're "wired" or under too much stress. See *Cable*.

WITCH   Ugly fearful part of self that needs to be changed. Manipulative, controlling; self-hating, loathing. Not seeing own inner beauty, the diamond inside. One must not use power to manipulate or mislead. There are karmic payments when one uses energy destructively instead of creatively.

WIZARD   See *Magician*.

WOLF   Ravenous desires, unfulfilled appetites; sly, sneaky. Attacks peace of mind and well being. Fill up from within; honor own selfhood.

WOMAN   See *Female*.

WOMB   Safety, security, nurturing with no responsibility. One may never return to the state of dependency without responsibility; but may recognize the security in creative power, and the loving protection of the divine, or God self within.

WOOD   Flexible, warm, nurturing, calming. When a part of the tree, represents aliveness that can be molded or shaped into new form.

WOOL   Soft, warm, nurturing.

WORLD   Reality you experience in space time awareness. Your own world; perceptions, beliefs, limitations. See *Earth*.

WORM   Aspects of self you prefer not to look at; those feeding on decay or negativity. Lack of awareness; lowly opinion of self. Earth worms prepare and enrich the soil; go ahead and start your planting. Recognize inner beauty.

WORSHIP   Acknowledging higher levels of consciousness; honoring the God within. Also, cutting self off from inner God, looking without to something or someone separate from yourself. One may worship many things which comes from a consciousness of separateness; only inner truth will lead you to fulfillment and wholeness.

WOUND   An imbalance from which energy is escaping; mental, emotional, physical. See where wound is located; what you are doing to harm yourself, dissipate your energy. Often reflects an emotional wound; you have not released someone or feel hurt and neglected. Forgive, let go, and return to your own creative center for fulfillment.

WREATH   Celebration of growth.

WRECK   Scattered energy, lack of awareness. If vehicle wreck, abrupt halt in direction; it is not necessary to do it the hard way. Car represents physical energy; boat = emotional; plane = spiritual and creative. You are sabotaging your goals. Get in touch with purpose; meditate, and plan accordingly.

WRITE   Communication, self-expression.

$\overline{X}$ **X-RAY**   Penetration, focused energy; electromagnetic radiation. Getting an inside look with more clarity. Look within; do not linger on the surface of things. Greater depth required for insight.

$\overline{Y}$ **YARD**   Growth, expression of self. Notice whether yard is neat, clean, has flowers, weeds, and so on.

YARN   Spinning a yarn. See *Weave, Thread.*

YAWN   Boredom; lack of energy, motivation.

YEAR   Unit of time; completion of growing and learning cycle. See *Numbers* (12) and *Time.*

YEAST   Ingredient within that causes growth and expansion. Rising to the occasion.

YELL   Pay attention; get attention, call for help.

YELLOW   Peace, harmony. If turning yellow, may indicate fear; lacking the courage of convictions.

YIN-YANG   The Chinese symbol for the dynamic union of opposites; secret of changes, life, death and regeneration in the universe. The yin principle is female, creative intuitive, receptive, dark, negative, body, the unconscious. The yang principle is male, intellect, strength, light, positive, spirit, consciousness. The polar energies are fully expressive in their unity or oneness. We must achieve a balance of the female-male energies within us to evolve from the earth plane. (Note: My guidance includes the creative-intuitive as a combined female energy. Most other systems put the creative under the male energy.) See *Female, Male.*

YOGA   Body, mind and spirit harmony; integration, unity. See *Meditation.*

YOKE   Harnessing of self to some belief or attitude that has obviously become a burden. Protection, focusing of energy and direction.

YOUNG   Openness, lighthearted, playful, creative part of self; few restrictions or limitations. Young at heart.

YO-YO   Going up and down emotionally; not learning lessons in experiences, repeating the same old patterns.

ZEBRA   Mixture of known and unknown, white and black, parts of self; balance in masculine and feminine energies. Paradoxes in your nature.

Z

ZEN   Path of intuition; spiritual discipline and meditation.

ZERO   See *Numbers.*

ZIP CODE   Address, identity, grounding; location or bearings. Add numbers to get meaning. See *Numbers.*

ZIPPER   Closing things in or opening things up.

ZODIAC   Principle of time; potential for expression and manifestation in time space. Culmination of all traits, aspects, potential within self. Balance within; earth, air, fire and water. See *Astrology, Horoscope.*

ZOMBIE   One no longer in touch with feelings, emotions; unable to function mentally, emotionally, spiritually. Blocking self from aliveness through fear. Lack of self love; low energy.

Loosen up and begin to get back in touch with the flow of life by crawling out of your grave. Join the ranks of the living. Fear is an illusion, and the only way to go is up.

ZOO   Different ways of expressing animal instincts within self that are restricted, caged. Seeing life as a zoo; many variations of physical, mental, emotional and spiritual energies. Remember to laugh at yourself and to be understanding, compassionate toward the many forms of self-expression. Also, your present situation is like a zoo; relax and enjoy.

Over 450 additional dream symbols.

If you haven't found the symbol
you're looking for in the
main glossary pages, look here.

ARCHIVES All souls have spiritual records that go with them from lifetime to lifetime. They show one's progress in terms of growth, consciousness, self-knowledge and self-love.

ARMOR Protection for the mind, body, and spirit.

ARTERY Either you are going with the flow or you have to slow down, relax and learn to turn it over.

ASSASSIN The "killing" off of elements no longer useful in your waking life. Now you can get on with the new.

AUTHORITY You always have a voice within showing you the way to achieve your best benefits. That's the authority within. All it takes is for you to listen to that voice and to trust your instincts.

AXIS Alignment with the universal order of things allowing you to maintain that all-important life-sustaining balance.

BACCANAL The over-expression of the 2nd chakra.

BACTERIA There are the bacteria that support life, and bacteria that tear it down. Both are necessary on this planet. Which type Seems more prevalent in your dream?

BAIL As in bailing water out of a boat--rescuing you emotionally--or bailing you out of jail--setting you free.

BALANCE To be on a steady keel and not at one extreme or the other. To be able to give and receive, love and be loved, work and play in perfect unison.

BALLAD A slow, meaningful, innate rhythmic pattern that allows for a harmonious existence.

BALONEY Either a nurturing food or perhaps you are feeding yourself a line of baloney.

BANDIT Your inner highwayman ripping yourself off. This is more easily done if your energy is down. Worry and fear are the bandit's best friends.

A

B

BANNISTER Your need to hold on to something. If you are ascending the stairs, you are going in the right direction, if descending, it can lead you to a loss of energy.

BAREFOOT A way to ground yourself.

BAR MITZVAH, BAT MITZVAH Becoming a Bar or Bat Mitzvah marks a time when a boy or girl is old enough to take on certain duties and responsibilities. If you are being so honored in your dream, it's saying that you are a responsible person. Mazel tov!

BARREL A barrel of fun. Or, not so good, being at the bottom of the barrel.

BASE The 'centered' part of you that ensures your mental, emotional, and spiritual stability.

BAT Unknown power that hasn't righted itself yet. Upside down!

BEAM Protective, energizing. Stay in the light at all times, especially when lessons seem difficult.

BEAST Fear is a beast, worry is a beast, and unhappiness is a beast. We create our own beasts and we can shoo them away.

BEATNIK The free, unconventional self. Daring to be you.

BEAUTIFUL See your own beauty and letting the vision lead you to self-esteem and self-love.

BENEFICIARY The recipient of God-given gifts. Make sure you are able to receive. Most people are givers, but to be balanced, you must also be able to accept that which is offered you.

BERSERK Low energy producing highly negative behavior.

BILLIONAIRE Having boundless energy.

BINGO Treat the ups and downs as a game and come out a winner.

BIOGRAPHY The most important biography that applies to you is the one that shows how much wisdom, self-love and self-knowledge you accumulate over this lifetime.

BIRTHDAY SUIT If you dream you are naked and in Macys window, you are merely stating "Here I am without pretensions or cover-ups. And additionally, I am not phony."

BISEXUAL Merging energy with an opposite sex or same sex partner.

BITCH A lack of self-love and self-respect that needs a mirror for these same negative qualities in order to feel okay.

BLACK MAGIC When an individual believes that the occult can affect him or her, the brain might follow that thought so as to create some negative patterns. Remember that nothing can influence you adversely unless you agree to it.

BLAZE Purification and renewal. The purpose of this is to clear out old thinking and to make room for a new beliefs and understanding.

BLISS The natural state that's inherent in all people if they will just let themselves feel it. Be happy, dammit!

BLOOPER Even in dreams, we make them. So the message is to forget that perfectionist side of yourself and laugh at the various mishaps bound to happen.

BOA CONSTRICTOR Facing one, you know your kundalini is on the rise.

BOLT Unlatch the door so that all good things can come through it.

BONANZA Multiple rewards for something well done.

BOND You are connected spiritually to your three guidance and your guardian angel. They are with you at all times.

BOOMERANG What you sow you reap. Work on your karmic ties.

BOOT   Need to get grounded and balanced.

BOSOM   Comforting, nurturing, maternal. Giving oneself solace.

BOUNDARY   Setting limits. Knowing what's right or wrong for you.

BREW   The story you have created for yourself.

BRICK   Something sturdy to build on for your spiritual quest. Also, that part of you that is strong and reliable and always there for you. "A brick."

BUZZER   Wake up! You may have been asleep during life's lessons.

C

CALISTHENICS   Building yourself up for a healthier life.

CAMELOT   Your own mythical setting. Your own castle of Peace, beauty and perfection.

CARNIVAL   All those parts of you in a fabulous, fun setting. If you see yourself on the Ferris wheel or on the carousel, however, perhaps you are going round and round in some situation or other.

CASH   Energy. Receiving cash in a dream means you are willing to accept abundance. If you are giving it away shows your willingness to share. But in all cases, giving and receiving should always be a 50/50 proposition. Otherwise you are out of balance.

CAST   All those characters on a stage? They're all you!

CAULDRON   Obviously you are cooking something up. Probably your strategy for spiritual enfoldment.

CAVALRY   Call out the troops. You need all the backup you can get.

CELESTIAL   Reaching for the stars. Be clear on what you want to achieve and what you want in life. It's all there waiting for you.

CENTER Balance, being able to stay calm in all circumstances.

CHAMPION In metaphysical terms, someone who is working on him or herself to achieve the gifts of intuitiveness, consciousness, self-love and self-knowledge.

CHANNEL Your intuitive powers enable you to get the answers you need to progress spiritually. Believe your gut reactions.

CHANT Verbal prayer. Communicating with your guidance.

CHAUFFEUR Sitting back and allowing that part that serves you take you on your journey.

CHERUB Your innocent child part spreading love everywhere within you.

CHIEF A version of you as someone leading your many selves in a wise and prudent fashion.

CHOREOGRAPHY The dance of life as choreographed by you—your needs and desires fulfilled with every step you take. If you have two left feet, you are too much in your head.

CINDERELLA An opportunity to get yourself from down under, to sparkle, to shine. It can be taken away from you but good fortune will always find you again.

CLEAVER Chopping away some stubborn part you yourself that just won't go away!

CLINIC Letting your inner healer work its magic.

CLOISTER Your protective retreat. Conversely, remaining cloistered can impede your spiritual growth.

COCAINE Clouding the brain, seeing things in a distorted way, falling victim to dependency, avoiding reality.

COCKPIT All the flying instruments right there before you, so now you can take off.

COCOON Your safe, inner environment. The place to go to when facing life's challenges.

COED   Your feminine creative self attending spiritual college for advanced studies in the art of self-realization.

COIFFURE   Determining the way you want to use your inner strength—hair is strength.

COITUS   Merging of the feminine creative and masculine assertive energies. Or the feminine/feminine or masculine/masculine as in same sex unions.

COLLAGE   Fitting together the various aspects of your life so that they work together as a whole.

COLLAR   The 5th chakra, located in the throat, needs the freedom to communicate freely.

COLLISION   You bumping into you. Best to step aside and let you pass, move on and grow.

COLOSSUS   The big, mighty self. Very powerful, but this power must be used responsibly and with positive goals in mind.

COLON   The route taken for that which needs to be let go of.

COMIC   A funny dream is saying "laugh at it all." And that you may be taking life far too seriously.

COMPANION   Your best companion is yourself, plus you have three guidance and one guardian angel that walk with you through life. God doesn't trust you here alone.

CONCEIVE   A fresh new 'you' being formed.

CONTAINER   A place to store your well-earned spiritual growth and consciousness.

CONVERTIBLE   If riding with the top down, you are open to what the universe has to offer you. The sky is the limit.

CONVOY   Your many selves on the move toward better understanding, attitudes, and behaviors.

CORD   Each night when dreaming, we leave the body by a silver cord. It takes you way out into the universe. When waking up, the silver cord is reeled in. Should the cord be severed, that's what is known as death, except there is no death...remember? It just means you get to go home.

CORSET Impedes your freedom and life force (breath), keeps you tied up.

CO-STAR You have many and they are all you—all co-starring with you in your movie or play. Get ready for your close-up.

COTTAGE You are the house you live in. If large, your energy and potential are large. If a cottage, you are comfortable with your rate of growth at this time. If a shack, well...

COSTUME A role you are playing that covers up your true identity.

COUNTERFEIT Might look like the real you but you know it isn't.

COUP DE GRACE Finishing off a part of you that is no longer needed.

COUPLES The two most significant sides of yourself experiencing life's lessons together.

COYOTE Unpredictable. An attack on your sensibilities at any time without warning. Also, howling at your lot in life.

CREVICE Watch where you step in any given situation. Be careful at the decisions you make.

CROTCH The center of your feminine creative and masculine assertive powers.

CROWD Your many selves all together.

CRYSTAL A symbol for clarity...being "crystal clear."

CUL DE SAC One-Way in, same way out. Can't move through.

CURE If ill in a dream, it merely means you are low on energy. Don't panic. Meditate instead. The best cure.

D   **DAREDEVIL**   Taking risks is part of life even if they don't work out. Congratulations for trying.

DATEBASE   Your spiritual circuitry that connects the conscious with the unconscious mind; your main workstation that deals with every aspect of your life.

D-DAY   A confrontation between your positive and negative attitudes and beliefs.

DECORATION   Recognition for a courageous act, no doubt in meeting a spiritual challenge. Also, beautifying your spiritual home.

DEMILITARIZE   Declaring a truce between your warring aspects.

DEMOLITION   The old way of thinking and believing is being dismantled so that the new can be installed.

DEPARTMENT   The soul has many departments in what could be termed the human Pentagon, so many, in fact, that it would be impossible to come up with a correct number.

DICTATOR   Your inner control freak.

DIVE   Uh-oh, going in the wrong direction, and in a hurry, too. Straighten up and fly right!

DIVINE   The ultimate state if higher consciousness.

DOCUMENT   Since everything in a dream is about you, a document testifies to your spiritual growth. It is an important record that will reflect how far you have come in your quest.

DOMINO EFFECT   Everything leads to something else, so pay attention to everything you initiate. Remember, it all begins with us, everything we do, say, or believe.

DRY   In danger of drying up. Pull up your energy and keep your fertile mind happy and healthy.

DUET   In harmony with another part of yourself to create serenity and joy.

DUST It can cover up your light. So grab a dust rag and make your surfaces shine.

DYNAMIC Either you've got energy that won't quit or you need to get it.

EASY When something appears easy in a dream, you know you are saving yourself some unnecessary strain.

E

EBOOK Your digital book of life.

EDGE At the point where you might to embark on something new in your life.

EFFEMINIATE Feminine creative chemistry that outbalances Masculine assertive energy.

EFFIGY Hanging oneself symbolically when dissatisfied with an action or actions.

EIGHT Money, power and prestige plus cosmic consciousness (knowing what's going on around you.) Having an 8 in a dream is rare...if you get one you know you are doing okay.

EJACULATE To provide a major energy proponent that creates new life.

ELECTROLYSIS The symbolic removal of one's minor strengths. Having one's head shaved would indicate complete strength Loss. Poor old Samson.

ELEVEN 11=2, so therefore the balance of the masculine assertive and the feminine creative. Also, balance of work/play and left brain/right brain. It should all be a balanced 50/50.

EMAIL Even your guidance is up to date when communicating with you.

EMASCULATE When a negative aspect of yourself attempts to remove your strong, masculine identity.

EMBARRASS   Too much concern over what others think of you or even what you think of yourself. If you've done something to embarrass yourself in a dream, it's just to tell you that you are only human.

EMBRYO   The creation of a new you.

EMPIRE   If earthly, it's not permanent. If spiritual, it's eternal.

ENCORE   Now that you did something great and to be proud of, can you do it again?

ENCYCLOPEDIA   You embody all the wisdom of the world. It's all within you.

ENNUI   Think your energy up and get out of the quicksand.

ENVELOPE   Is there a message inside? If not, you might not be ready for the message at this time.

EPIDEMIC   Need to upgrade your immune system to protect your mind, body and spirit.

EQUILIBRIUM   The proper balancing of the body, mind, spirit. If one element is off, the other two are likewise.

ERASER   Rub out that which no longer serves you.

ERECTION   Masculine symbol ready to exercise its function.

ESP   Intuition. Accessing thoughts and visions of a higher order. A pre-cognitive dream is an example.

ETERNAL   That's life! There has never been a time when your soul did not exist and there will never be a time when your soul doesn't exist.

ETHNIC   By the time you reach your 23rd and final incarnation on this earth plane, you will have experienced multiple races and religions. So you cannot judge another person's ethnicity because you have probably been it yourself.

EXAMINATION   Looking within to view your spiritual worth. Also, you are studying for a spiritual test

EXCAVATION   Digging up the past. Why bother? Live for today!

EXCOMMUNICATE   Reconnect with your highest good, let nothing cut you off.

EXHAUSTION   Time for renewal, rest, introspection, meditation, self-love. Forgiveness, and connecting with all your positive outlets possible.

EXODUS   Walking away from troubling influences.

EYELID   Open your eyes. Look around and be conscious of your world.

FABLE   You are the weaver if tales. Your story reads like somebody lived it. Somebody did. You!

F

FADE-IN   Seeing gradually what's really important—it all becomes clear, coming into focus.

FADE-OUT   Completion of a scene in your life. It's like riding into the sunset. Getting ready for a new day.

FAIL   A dream that depicts failure of any sort is a teaching dream advising that failure is impossible. Trade the word for "growth.

FAITH   Go for it. know that you are held in great esteem by your guidance. Now you must match that support by having faith in yourself and the great universe.

FASHION   The many roles we play in life. Each outfit reflects some aspect of your many selves and what they represent.

FELATIO   Extracting the powerful masculine life-giving force.

FELON   The need to imprison your criminal aspect so as to protect all your other aspects.

FIG LEAF   Keeping your masculine assertive or feminine creative identities under wraps.

FILE CABINET   Where the records of your lives are kept.

FIRE EXTINGUISHER   Putting out one's flame of life. Keep your energy high and the flame cannot be extinguished.

FIRST AID   Heal thyself. You have everything in your spiritual first aid kit to do it.

FIVE   Change. If something isn't working, you have the power to change it.

FLAK   Hey, someone's shooting at you as you reach the heights on your fabulous spiritual journey. Could be you.

FLOCK   All the parts of yourself that identify with one another.

FLOW   Go with it!

FORCE   Life and the power to keep it going.

FOREPLAY   Another aspect of the energy exchange within you.

FOUR   The one-to-one relationship. All souls must, in one lifetime or another, feel the ecstasy of exchanging energy with a significant other. If in a relationship or marriage without heart-to-heart gratification, it is not s true union.

FRAGRANCE   The essence of spiritual consciousness and growth.

FRATERNITY   A get-together of your masculine aspects. A sorority would be the female equivalent.

FREE WILL   Everything up to the age of 28 is destined. After the age of 28, we are given free will to choose how we want to move toward spiritual enlightenment.

FROST   Chilled emotions.

FUMIGATE   Making life fresh again.

FURLOUGH   Taking a break from all those lessons and tests. Did you know you can request a break now and then? Just ask.

FUTURE   There will always be one, there has always been one. We conceive of beginnings and endings...the future has no ending.

GANGPLANK Stepping from one safe place to another without falling into the emotions.

GEEK In your head, maybe too much. Excess left-brain thinking.

GHOST TOWN What used to be and is no longer. Make sure you are not living in one.

GIVING AND RECEIVING Necessary balance of the two. Giving is easier for most people. They don't want to feel beholden by receiving. But knowing how to receive is vital so as to avoid "having" learn this lesson in later life, perhaps in a nursing facility. Learn to give and take in balance.

GLITTER A test for you to discern between what's real and what isn't. Remember, all that glitters isn't gold.

GNOSTIC Pertaining to your personal spiritual record in conjunction with the laws of the universe. All records are kept and stored, to be reviewed later by your guidance.

GORILLA Mighty, but not fully cognizant. Brawn, not brain.

GOSPEL SINGER Harmony and appreciation for all that is given and received.

GRAB BAG Not knowing what lies ahead. Taking what you get out of life and running with it.

GRAMMAR SCHOOL On the way to full consciousness.

GRAPES If purple, the highest spiritual plain. If green, growth and consciousness. Either way, you can't lose.

GRAVY Added value to your life, but it doesn't hurt to check underneath to see what's really there.

GREENHOUSE Cultivating and nurturing a pattern of growth and enlightenment.

GREEN LIGHT There's no stopping you...

GROIN The central balance point for either masculine assertive or feminine creative energy.

GROUND   The foundation needed for true balance and rationality.

GROWTH   Working on oneself in terms of body, mind, and spirit. Moving from one lesson to the next while accumulating the wisdom you will take with you after this incarnation.

GYNOCOLOGIST   Might be a sign to go see one. Otherwise, know thy uterus.

H   **HAG**   The self-neglected female creative persona.

HAVEN   Safety, security, and peace of mind.

HAZE   Mental cloudiness, not seeing clearly or ahead. Low energy.

HELP   You are never without it. You have three guides who walk with you through life. If in need, ask and you will receive.

HETEROSEXUAL   Leaning heavily on either the masculine assertive side or the feminine creative.

HIBERNATE   Going within, allowing energy to go dormant, mainly in the winter months.

HIT AND RUN   Injury to oneself followed by denial.

HITCH HIKE   Not moving under your own steam, dependence on others.

HOBO   Poverty of body, mind, spirit.

HONEY   Your sweet nature but you can get sticky about things.

HOOFER   Dancing to your own tune.

HUMAN   The current vehicle that houses the soul that has always existed and will always exist.

HUNDRED   100 = 1 or 10. If a 1, a new beginning. If a 10, new beginnings with experience. Those in their 23rd or final lifetimes on this planet will be in the latter category, more intuitive, more willing to work on their issues.

HUSBAND A mate for your feminine creative even if you are male.

HUSH In a dream means silent yourself and listen. Also, rethink what you were about to say. Most turmoil on this planet begins with the spoken word.

HYDROFOIL Gliding over the emotions, not letting things bother you. Not sinking when there are problems.

ICE AGE Frozen emotions. Thaw out already!

ICON Paying homage to an exalted part of yourself.

IGNITE A burst of energy. Some individuals have what is known as charisma, which can ignite and raise the energy levels of themselves and others so that they have the sensation that they are flying.

ILLUMINATE The aura of bright white light surrounding you when fueled by energy. The more energy you put out, the brighter your aura.

IMMATURE Refusing to leave that safe, comfy place called childhood.

IMMIGRANT Foreign aspect of the self.

IMPEACH If you are being impeached in a dream, see where your integrity has been compromised in waking life.

INCOME TAX Your energy being taken from you. Any tax will do that.

INNER EAR Listen and really get the message.

INTERVENE The wisdom to de-fuse a potentially explosive disaster. Or to voice and opinion that might improve the outcome of a certain situation. Or to place yourself between two opposing factions.

INTRICATE Something requiring close study in order to see its inner workings.

INTROVERT More interested in lone pursuits of quality rather than senseless group activity. Finding your answers through studied introspection and going within.

INTUITION Your God-given ability to discern the nature of the universe through your own cosmic powers. Having the eyes to see and the ears to hear; trusting one's own gut for answers.

I.O.U. The putting off of karmic debt that will have to be paid.

ITINERARY The many stops along on your spiritual path as you travel along, the first 28 years having already been decided. After 28, you have free will to choose how you want things to go.

J **JACUZZI** Being in the emotions, but at least it's fun and refreshing.

JAMBOREE All your joyous voices giving a magnificent performance.

JANITOR Maintaining a clean mental, physical, and spiritual state of mind. Also we have to clean up any messes we have made. Sometimes, we feel we have to clean up messes that others have made, but keep in mind, codependency is not healthy.

JAVELIN Extending your reach to the stars. There's so much out there for you...

JET Major movement in your spiritual life that keeps you flying at an accelerated speed.

JIGSAW PUZZLE Putting all the pieces together to make a whole picture. Don't act until all the evidence is there.

JOCKEY Hang on. The ride is often hazardous.

JOKE When you think about it, so much that happens in life is funny, so laugh at it all. Also, if you are taking yourself too seriously, that's no joke.

JUICE You might have to squeeze to get what you want. But don't squeeze the life out of the situation.

K **KABOB** Getting skewered.

KALEIDISCOPE Letting all the pieces fall into place to make a beautiful picture.

KEYPAD Making all your metaphysical connections easily and effortlessly.

KICK Energy sometimes aimed where you most need it. Also, getting a kick out of life.

KIDNEY What clearer symbol for letting go toxicity in yourself and in relationships.

KINFOLK You, you, you, you, and you.

KLUTZ Treating everyday mishaps with comic relief. It's okay to laugh at yourself. In fact, it's necessary.

KUDOS Appreciating you for your earnest desire to become fully conscious, to love who you are and what you stand for, and to know as much as possible about the magnificent spirit that you are.

LAVENDER The yin-yang balance of the feminine creative. The agility to go within and to increase consciousness.

L

LAZY Lacking in motivation due to decreased energy. Perhaps thinking "why bother?" But everyone has a purpose in life. Yours is probably right before your eyes.

LEAK The drip, drip, drip of emotions slowly creeping up on you.

LEISURE Time off for good behavior without tests and lessons.

LESSON What we need in order to grow. They come upon us in an endless stream. Let them come and know that you chose to be in the classroom.

LEVEE An emotional boundary so as not to overwhelm you.

LIP The dream might be telling you that giving your opinion when none is ask can be dangerous. Or that giving your opinion when you *are* asked can *also* be dangerous.

LOCOMOTIVE All aboard! You're on your way. The locomotive reflects the power within you to move and move fast.

LULLABY The harmony of innocence lulling the child part inside you into a place of security and peace.

LUST An active 2nd chakra seeking release. May not be taking responsibility for the consequences.

LYRIC It's your song; you wrote the words. Probably the melody, too.

M **MAGIC** In a dream, creating a world of awe and wonder around you. You are the magician. You are the creator.

MEDAL It's better to get a medal in the dream state than in your waking life because it comes to you from your guidance. Look closely at what it says on the back. For example, it might read: For your courage and willingness to expand your consciousness.

MELONCHOLY Sadness brought on by low energy. Get your energy up by meditating daily and you probably won't have that dream—or that feeling--again.

MERCY The state of mind that provides compassion for you and for others.

METAMORPHISIS The change that occurs when you go from an ego-based life to one that is spiritually charged.

METEOR Seeing one while dreaming means here is such a thing known as "meteoric" success. Let it be yours.

MICROSCOPE Look closely; you'll see things about your life that you didn't detect with the naked eye.

MIMIC Find your own voice. You can't live your own life until you do.

MISSION A prime question for all: What is your purpose? What are you on earth to do?

MORTAL Mortality is a myth. The soul never dies. It is immortal.

N **NEIGHBOR** Your next door you.

NERD Possibly using too much of the left brain to be properly balanced.

NINE Completion. Learning your lessons. Moving on.

NOMAD That dessert-dweller within you thirsting for new vistas. You can't grow if you are static.

NOOSE The ultimate inability to communicate. Pay attention to what is happening in your fifth chakra--the seat of self-expression. If you are suppressing your emotions, do yourself a favor and speak your peace.

NOSEBLEED Leaking energy.

OBESE An over-nourished persona, not in balance. $\overline{O}$

OATH A sacred agreement you made with yourself and your

OPEN DOOR Entering a new phase in your quest for awareness, moving forward, discovering what lies beyond.

ORBIT If you have the eyes to see and the ears to hear, you are in true orbit.

OUTLAW Running from oneself.

OXYGEN The elixir of life. If you are wearing an oxygen mask, you need to relax, breathe, and let stress melt away.

PACIFIER A primal need for nurturing. $\overline{P}$

PACK RAT A pack rat in your dreams speaks of an impoverished soul. Never having enough. Hoarding as a way to quell poverty thinking. The more junk you have, the safer you may feel, but it's alse security. You can also be a mental pack rat, storing away useless information, or an emotional pack rat, with a collection of grudges and grievances. An all-around decluttering is called for.

PALLBEARER Carrying the weight of a dead part of yourself that needs to be buried. As miraculous beings, we shed old parts of ourselves regularly, parts that were once alive with usefulness but have now served their purpose and are obsolete. The time has come to move on so that we can cultivate and learn from our current inner teachers. And to finally bury the past.

PATIENT Healing yourself. Also, being patient. Allowing time to bring about the best solution.

PHOBIA An irrational fear or so it appears on the surface, but possibly originating in a former incarnation and borne out of an unpleasant experience. Look at what scares you in a dream.

PORNOGRAPHY A substitute for a functioning 2nd chakra. Might be based on fear of intimacy or commitment.

POWER An innate force that can be used positively or negatively. Might be associated with an out of control ego.

POWER OUTAGE A temporary energy failure that impedes the carrying out of your needs.

PREDATOR 2nd chakra-fixation targeting the child within.

PRETZEL Twisting yourself out of shape.

PRIMA DONNA The insecure self, operating out of low self-esteem and, at the same time, the delusion of grandeur. The inflated ego is at work here.

PROFESSOR The wise teacher that resides in all of us. If a student, listen attentively.

PROM Celebration after having completed many lessons and having passed many tests.

PROMISCUITY The part of oneself that has trouble being faithful to oneself.

PROSPERITY Your financial status in a dream reflects the quality of your life. Your God-given right to abundance, sometimes tempered with a fear of success. You get exactly out of life what you think you deserve, nothing more, nothing less.

PUBERTY The blossoming of the new stage in your spiritual development.

PUPIL Life is school with many spiritual tests to pass. Knowing and loving oneself is key to getting a good grade from one's guidance. It is the most important test in the curriculum. If you are having trouble accepting yourself, you may be getting poor grades in your "dream" schoolwork.

QUACK Watch out for the quack persona in in oneself. That which may not be exhibiting the highest degree of integrity.

QUAKER In a dream state, this is the ability to still the mind and to speak only when the spirit within moves you.

QUARANTINE Keeping confined any negatives may be you putting out so that they don't spread to the rest of your qualities.

QUESTION You can ask any question you like and then wait for the answer in a dream. Best to jot the question down before going to sleep and then to decipher the dream upon awakening. Then look the key points in this very same dream book.

QUIET Communion with God. You can't have this special time with a racket going on.

RAPIDS When a person's emotional life being tossed this way and that, grounding is needed.

REBEL Taking a stand--refusing what isn't right for you--trusting your intuition. Choosing your battles.

REHAB The attempted un-doing of harm done to the body, mind, and spirit through negative thought and action.

RED CROSS Your own innate healing station.

REHEARSAL Reviewing all you've learned spiritually before the big examination.

RELAPSE Dreams chart your progress and also show you where you may have slipped. Pay close attention and remedy the situation.

RETRO If living in the past, you could be missing out on what's happening now.

RHYTHM What's the tempo of the dream? Fast, slow? That will give you some indication of your speed in acquiring full consciousness.

RUBBLE Rebuilding one's existence. As the song goes: Take a deep breath, pick yourself up, dust yourself off, and start all over again.

S **SADNESS** A scenario in which you are sad shows your energy has diminished. Get your energy up high again and you won't have such a dream.

SAFETY Security that comes from within. Knowing that your guidance watches over you at all times.

SALT A symbol reflecting your spiritual worthiness. The phrase "Salt of the Earth" comes to mind.

SCHOOL BUS The vehicle delivering you to the schoolroom of life. You will be the driver and all the students. Your guidance will be your teachers.

SCORE If you see a scorecard, what's are your marks? Your guidance is writing it all down for you.

SEISMOGRAPH Perhaps you are on shaky ground...need to get your emotional bearings.

SEVEN There are those who consider it lucky to see a seven in a dream. They're right. It is a lucky number as well as a mystical one. For balance, 7 refers to the alignment of the chakras. And finally, it's the number that indicated going within to find the answers to life's many puzzles.

SHINE The brightness that vibrates from you in waves, attracting others. Charisma. Laughing. Joyful. A happy dream will speak volumes about your "shine" quotient. So will an unhappy dream. However, all dreams are positive—giving you valuable information.

SILK Smooth to the touch, it reflects how your life is progressing. Other fabrics in a dream will determine if things are tough—burlap, for instance. Or just humdrum such as cotton. Nylon alludes to artificiality.

SMART PHONE In a dream, using your smart phone is a smart way to send and receive messages from your guidance.

SMILE Lighting up the positive circuitry and energy of your being. Becoming a beacon of light for others.

SOUL When you have 'soul,' your have compassion and love for oneself and others.

SPEEDBUMP Caution on your journey, going too fast, being too anxious. Take your time.

SPIRIT The universal force that sweeps through you. The human spirit cannot be dampened except when the flow of natural energy ceases. Meditation on a daily basis will prevent this from happening. Even when the road is rough, meditation will enliven the spirit and the day will be better.

SUPERMAN If this popular icon should pop up in a dream, know it is you in tights and that you can fly to heights you never thought possible.

SWASTIKA Recognition of the supreme cosmos as interpreted in ancient times. However, it has been a misused symbol used by tyrants, so look to see if your control issues are in check.

TANTRA Becoming one. The ultimate merging of energies embodied in the masculine assertive and the feminine creative.

TAROT A way of divining your future in a medium that rules out coincidence. But the reading of the cards have no power over you. Take what you like and leave the rest.

TAXI Giving permission to a part of yourself to temporarily be in charge of your life. Don't forget the tip.

TEENAGER The unformed, searching, insecure self that must experience this stage of life in order to emerge as a mature being.

TELLER Dispensing to you the energy you have put in a place for safekeeping. Taking this energy as needed or depositing it for later use.

TENTACLE   Your influence is far-reaching. You have the power to grab what you want and what you need.

TITANIC   In a dangerous emotional situation. Make sure your mental, physical, and spiritual lifeboats are in good repair.

TOLLBOOTH   Stop and pay your karma. Even if you have use of Fasttrack.

TORPEDO   Self-destructive behavior armed, aimed, and fired at yourself when you are in a vulnerable emotional state.

TOUPEE   A source of artificial strength—having the appearance of the real thing (hair), but not the genuine quality.

TRANSEXUAL   The transition necessary to manifest one's true identity.

TRICYCLE   A first attempt to get balance in life.

TWITTER   Short bursts of information and communication for the self.

TYRANT   The control freak within.

U

UNDERTOE   Watch where you tread when in an emotional state to avoid being sucked under.

UNEXPECTED   In the dream state, scenarios occur that surprise you. Whatever the vision, there is an important message attached.

UNISEX   Revealing the masculine assertive and the feminine creative aspects as equal.

UNIVERSE   The mysterious vastness that you are so much a part of You are the universe. You are made up of the same elemental structure as the rest of the cosmos and you embody the same energy.

V

VALEDICTORIAN   Top of the class and, in fact, leading the class.

VALENTINE'S DAY   Make yourself your sweetheart.

VALUABLES Showing you that the only real treasure is the spiritual wisdom you take from your earthly tenure. Of most importance are the self-love and the self-knowledge you have achieved.

VASECTOMY Denying the creation of a new part of yourself.

VENTRILOQUIST Are you behaving like a puppet? Letting other voices, thoughts, actions come through you, provided by a different and separate source? Time to "get a life."

VISA The freedom to explore your many fascinating facets. Your passport to a richer, more rewarding life.

VOCAL Get it out, talk, expand, don't stuff. You weren't given a voice for nothing. If a vocalist, you are spreading harmony.

VOICEMAIL Incoming or outgoing messages from yourself.

WANDERER Moving from one stage of growth to another, from one lesson to another, from one test to another. Always searching for the answers that will take you to the apex of consciousness.

WARGAME The war within you that has you playing with destruction.

WARRANTY You come with one. The only requirement is that you learn your lessons before it runs out.

WASH BASIN What needs cleaning up? Also applicable to washing machine, wash cloth, soap, etc.

WEIGHTLIFTER Dealing with the weight of the world on your shoulders. Or a reminder to strengthen yourself.

WHIRLPOOL Something outside yourself dragging you 'round and 'round.

WHODUNNIT Just accept that it was you "whodunit." It all starts and continues with us. Look back and you will see where you instigated the events, dramas, battles, and even the really good times in your life.

WIMP Get a grip, unleash your extraordinary powers.

WINDBREAKER   Protection for the upper chakras.

WINDFALL   A great, unexpected supply of energy. You probably need it.

WIRETAP   A ploy to find out what's *really* going on with you. Don't be afraid of eavesdropping.

WORD PROCESSOR   Self expression made easy.

WORLD WAR   All your aspects in armed combat. Calm down, don't react, get your peacemaker aspect out there negotiating for an inner world without turmoil.

WORRY   The fastest possible way to deplete your energy.

WRESTLER   Putting yourself in an emotional headlock you may not be able to get out of.

WRONG MOVE   There are no wrong moves. There are only lessons to be learned.

X   **XEROX**   Copying the positive actions that have benefitted you.

XMAS   If you see this abbreviation in a dream, perhaps you should abbreviate all that credit card debt you are liable to build up.

X-RATED   The merging of masculine and feminine energies can get a bit steamy.

Y   **YACHT**   If you are travelling through an emotional patch, may as well do it in style. You are the boat...better to have all the accouterments rather than rough it in a dinghy.

YARMULKE   Spiritual head gear reminding you to keep up all spiritual work.

Z   **ZEBRA**   Seeing things in both black and white.

ZIGZAG   If you move in an irregular pattern, you make a lousy target.

Notes

Notes

Notes

Notes